DO YOU KNOW . . .

- Certain vegetables can *cause* calcification, inflammation, and pain in the joints
- Gout sufferers should NOT take vitamin C
- Victims of osteoarthritis risk additional pain if they use a popular artificial sweetener
- Garlic can control arthritis symptoms
- Daily massage can help children with arthritis, asthma, and diabetes
- Food allergies commonly aggravate rheumatoid arthritis

PLUS NATURAL ALTERNATIVES TO TREAT JUVENILE RHEUMATOID ARTHRITIS, SYSTEMIC LUPUS ERYTHEMATOSUS, ANKYLOSING SPONDYLITIS, BURSITIS, AND CARPAL TUNNEL SYNDROME

THE DELL NATURAL MEDICINE LIBRARY

PREVENTION, HEALING, SYMPTOM RELIEF . . . FROM NATURE TO YOU

Also Available from the Dell Natural Medicine Library:

NATURAL MEDICINE FOR HEART DISEASE

NATURAL MEDICINE FOR BREAST CANCER

NATURAL MEDICINE FOR BACK PAIN

NATURAL MEDICINE FOR DIABETES

THE DELL
NATURAL MEDICINE LIBRARY

NATURAL MEDICINE FOR
ARTHRITIS

Winifred Conkling

Foreword by Andrea D. Sullivan, PhD, ND, DHANP

A Lynn Sonberg Book

A Dell Book

Published by
Dell Publishing
a division of
Bantam Doubleday Dell Publishing Group, Inc.
1540 Broadway
New York, New York 10036

Grateful acknowledgment is made for permission to reproduce the illustrations courtesy of The Arthritis Foundation.

Copyright © 1996 by Lynn Sonberg Associates

The trademark Dell® is registered in the U.S. Patent and Trademark Office.

ISBN: 0-440-22169-2

Published by arrangement with Lynn Sonberg Book Associates

Printed in the United States of America

Published simultaneously in Canada

June 1997

10   9   8   7   6   5   4   3

OPM

For Bill and Nancy Prigg,
with love

ACKNOWLEDGMENTS

For their time and guidance, special thanks to Phoebe Reeve, herbalist, AHG, American Herbalist Guild Council Member, 1996; Jonathan Shore, MD, Diplomate of Homeotherapeutics, Member of Faculty of Homeopathy; and Andrea D. Sullivan, PhD, ND, Diplomate of the Homeopathic Academy of Naturopathic Physicians.

CONTENTS

FOREWORD

Arthritis is the nation's number-one crippling disease. More than 37 million Americans—one out of every seven people—have been diagnosed with the disease. If you include in the estimate those people who have experienced joint pain but have not been told by a doctor that they have arthritis, the number climbs to nearly 70 million.

Many arthritis sufferers turn to painkillers and antiinflammatory drugs to control their symptoms. All drugs have many effects; pain relief may be one effect, and gastrointestinal upset or a skin rash may be another unintended effect. Many of the drugs commonly used to treat arthritis can actually promote joint damage. These drugs mask the symptoms, which can make the patient feel better temporarily, but they do nothing to manage the underlying disease.

Fortunately there is another way.

Natural approaches to treating arthritis offer nontoxic ways of both easing the pain and improving the condition of the joints. Natural medicine should be thought of as complementary medicine, not alternative medicine. It is not in conflict or competition with conventional medicine; there are roles for both approaches in the healing process. Of course there are times when drugs and surgery are necessary, but these approaches should be chosen only after less intrusive, more natural methods have been tried.

Many senior citizens are particularly responsive to the natural approach to healing. The approach makes sense, and many older people remember the herbs and folk remedies their mothers or grandmothers may have used to manage arthritis or other illnesses. In addition many people with arthritis have grown tired of taking ten or twelve different pills every day, some just to control the negative effects of other drugs they're taking. All this medication can be confusing and potentially dangerous. Many people find natural medicine appealing because it can cut back on the number of medicines they must take.

Natural medicine involves treating the person, not just the disease. When someone walks into my office with arthritis, as a naturopath I don't see a case of arthritis, I see a person who happens to have arthritis. There are a number of factors that contribute to the disease, and it is my goal to understand my patient and design an approach to healing that will take into account that person's lifestyle and habits, as well as emotional issues and stresses. It cannot be overstated that as a naturopath I must understand my patients and the issues they face in their daily lives. Sometimes I can see that the arthritis began right after a divorce or right after a parent died, and I know that these stresses contributed to the progression of the disease.

Because the specific recommendations rely on the individual needs of the patient, there is no single natural remedy for arthritis. Every patient is different, and every patient needs a customized approach to healing that meets his or her specific needs and situation. After I understand my patient, I can begin to design a program for that individual that includes herbal treatments, a homeopathic remedy, nutritional counseling, massage, stress-reduction techniques, and exercise. The treatments suggested depend entirely on the needs and preferences of the individual patient.

Of course there are no guarantees—not every illness can be cured—but there are almost always things an individual can do either to halt the progression of most forms of arthritis or to reduce the limitations imposed by the disease. By making certain changes in lifestyle and routine, most people with arthritis can make important strides toward feeling better and improving their overall health, even if the arthritis symptoms persist.

For the reader unfamiliar with natural healing, *Natural Medicine for Arthritis* does an excellent job of introducing the basic approaches of complementary medicine. This comprehensive volume covers the importance of diet, vitamin and mineral supplements, exercise, herbs, homeopathic remedies, acupressure, and stress reduction in the management of arthritis. In addition, the resource sections at the end of most chapters provide the reader with all the information necessary to find appropriate, qualified practitioners of natural healing to help in the journey toward health.

With an open mind and this book in hand, you can begin to discover a natural approach to managing your arthritis. This book is not intended to be a substitute for professional medical care; consult your physician or other qualified health practitioner before implementing the approaches to health care suggested in this book. Though you sometimes may feel that your body is the enemy, keep in mind that your body is striving to heal itself. By practicing the techniques of natural healing, you can help your body in its quest to conquer and overcome arthritis pain.

—ANDREA D. SULLIVAN, PhD, ND, DHANP

INTRODUCTION

Modern medicine deserves our respect. Advances in medical science and our understanding of disease have allowed people to live longer—and often better—than ever before. Simple infections that used to kill can now be controlled with antibiotics. Surgeons who once used unsophisticated instruments to perform crude procedures can now perform amazing feats in the operating room, removing cancerous tumors from the brain, rebuilding the valves of the heart, and replacing arthritic joints with synthetic versions that smoothly glide through a full range of motion.

Despite the progress there are still times when old-fashioned natural treatments can be more effective and less dangerous than breakthrough medical procedures. The methods of natural healing seem particularly well suited to chronic illnesses, such as arthritis, which can cause pain and discomfort for decades.

Natural medicine does not challenge medical orthodoxy. In fact natural medicine complements conventional medicine. The approach does not rule out the appropriate use of synthetic drugs and surgery, but focuses on the use of diet, nutritional supplements, exercise, herbs, acupressure, homeopathy, and mind-body techniques to manage the arthritis before such drastic measures are taken. There is a time and place for both approaches to health. As a person with arthritis, you can embrace and experiment with both conventional and natural methods of healing.

In recent years natural medicine has gone mainstream. Practices that would have been classified as quackery not long ago are now embraced by both patients and medical experts. Medical organizations that once ridiculed natural medicine now endorse many of the same recommendations that practitioners of natural medicine have been making for decades. For example naturopaths have long recommended that people eat a high-fiber diet, exercise regularly, reduce stress, and cut back on the consumption of fats, refined sugars, and food additives. Now most conventional practitioners recognize the wisdom of these suggestions.

In addition herbal remedies, acupressure, and other natural methods of healing have been incorporated into the curriculum and practice at many medical schools and hospitals. Even the conservative National Institutes of Health opened an Office of Alternative Medicine in 1993 and began funding research on various alternative-medicine techniques.

Natural medicine has also won the support and confidence of a growing number of Americans. According to a 1993 article in the *New England Journal of Medicine,* fully one out of three people used an alternative therapy within the last year, and more than 80 percent of those people used conventional medicine at the same time.

Natural Medicine for Arthritis offers arthritis sufferers a comprehensive guide to understanding the disease, as well as natural methods of dealing with it. The book introduces the concepts and theories behind natural medicine and offers concrete advice on steps to take to relieve arthritis symptoms. In addition *Natural Medicine for Arthritis* provides a thorough list of resources and organizations that can provide additional information and expertise in a number of areas.

When certain precautions are followed, natural medicine is safe and effective. Before trying any of the natural remedies described in this book, consult your health care providers, especially if you are under the care of a physician for a specific medical condition. Of course if you try a natural remedy and your condition becomes worse, discontinue treatment and seek professional help, either from your regular doctor or from a qualified naturopath, herbalist, homeopath, acupressurist, or other practitioner of natural medicine.

CHAPTER ONE

Understanding and Diagnosing Arthritis

Though most of us take them for granted, our joints allow us to climb out of bed in the morning and to perform countless motions—both mundane and magnificent—throughout the day. For most people these hinges of the human body glide effortlessly through their full range of motion, but for the nearly 40 million Americans with arthritis, movement means stiffness and sometimes excruciating pain.

Arthritis, a term that means "joint inflammation," actually refers to more than one hundred different diseases and disorders. In many cases the problem affects the *synovial joint,* a gel-filled capsule consisting of connective tissue that attaches one bone to another in a way that allows movement. To create a smooth hinge between the bones, cartilage covers the ends of the bones, and a membrane inside the joint secretes a lubricating gel known as synovial fluid. An outer shell or joint capsule surrounds the various components of the joint and keeps them intact. This system works remarkably well. In a healthy joint the bones glide back and forth and allow movement without grinding or rubbing bone against bone.

In a person with arthritis, however, the joint has become

damaged or diseased. There may not be enough synovial fluid in the joint, causing stiffness, or there may be too much, causing swelling around the joint. If the cartilage at the ends of the bones has worn or chipped away, bone may scrape against bone, causing additional pain.

Such cases of arthritis and joint deterioration can be caused by a hereditary condition or by injury, overuse, infection, or autoimmune disease. Poor circulation, an unbalanced diet, and lack of exercise can also result in joint inflammation.

In addition highly reactive molecules known as free radicals (or pro-oxidants) can bind to and destroy the cells, causing osteoarthritis, as well as other health problems. The body produces free radicals during metabolism, but antioxidants found in plant foods can protect against free-radical damage. Foods rich in vitamins C and E, beta-carotene, and selenium are particularly beneficial.

What Type of Arthritis Do You Have?

Since each type of arthritis demands a different treatment, the first step toward managing the pain is diagnosing the type of arthritis you have. Following are the major types of arthritis.

Osteoarthritis

Osteoarthritis, the most common type of arthritis, is often referred to as degenerative joint disease because it involves breakdown of the cartilage and bone in the joints, especially the joints of the fingers, hips, knees, and spine. Osteoarthritis afflicts to some degree approximately 40 million Americans, including 80 to 90 percent of people over age fifty and almost everyone over age sixty. While many older people write off the symptoms to the inevitable aches and pains of aging,

16 million Americans experience pain severe enough to compromise their joint function.

In most cases decades of wear and tear gradually damage the cartilage in the joints, causing it to harden and form bone spurs inside the joints. This cartilage breakdown causes the pain, inflammation, deformity, and restriction in range of motion characteristic of osteoarthritis.

Unlike other types of arthritis, which can strike suddenly, osteoarthritis usually takes its toll gradually, with the symptoms becoming worse over a number of years. Common warning signs of osteoarthritis include the following:

- Joint stiffness, especially in the mornings upon waking and after long periods of rest
- Joint tenderness and slight swelling (inflammation is not common with osteoarthritis)
- Cracking and creaking joints
- Loss of range of motion
- Pain when the joint is used

Primary osteoarthritis refers to degeneration caused by fifty to sixty years of joint use. In such cases there has been no single episode of joint injury; instead constant use, especially of the weight-bearing joints, has gradually eroded the cartilage in the joint. As we age, we must not only confront the cumulative damage of a lifetime of joint use, but the body also becomes less efficient at producing the enzymes used to manufacture and repair the cartilage. In other words our cartilage breaks down and our bodies fall behind in the ability to repair it.

Secondary osteoarthritis involves joint degeneration caused by inherited physical abnormalities in the joint, injury or trauma, or earlier joint disease, such as gout or rheumatoid arthritis. The previous condition leaves the cartilage either damaged or prone to damage, which then results in the symptoms of osteoarthritis.

While physical forces tear the joint apart, the body is hard

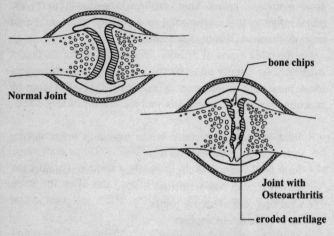

Normal Joint

bone chips

Joint with Osteoarthritis

eroded cartilage

Courtesy of Arthritis Foundation

at work trying to repair itself. In many cases, joint degeneration of osteoarthritis can be stopped or reversed by enhancing the function of the joint, which can be accomplished through many of the techniques of natural healing.

Osteoarthritis is often diagnosed by X rays, which show that the gap between the bones has narrowed or disappeared. Another sign is the appearance of bony nodes on the fingertip joints. Blood tests can't be used to confirm the diagnosis of osteoarthritis, but they can rule out several other types of arthritis and joint disease.

Rheumatoid Arthritis

Rheumatoid arthritis affects the entire body, causing chronic inflammation of many joints, as well as the skin, muscles, blood vessels, and in rare cases organs such as the heart and lungs. This serious condition plagues about 7 million Americans, about three fourths of them women. If improperly treated, rheumatoid arthritis can lead to joint deformity.

The disease causes the synovial membrane in the joints to divide and expand, causing inflammation and a buildup of joint fluid. Increased blood flow to the joints can cause redness and warmth.

Rheumatoid arthritis, which usually appears at age thirty-five to forty-five, typically manifests itself first as pain when moving a joint, especially in the early morning. The disease usually strikes the wrists and knuckles, and often the knee and the ball of the foot, though it can affect any joint in the body.

In addition to joint problems, rheumatoid arthritis can cause fever, fatigue, weight loss, anemia, and tingling hands and feet. If the organs become involved, complications can include an enlarged spleen, irregular heartbeat, or pleurisy, an inflammation of the membrane lining the lungs. Lumps (called rheumatoid nodules) can also appear in the joints, especially in the elbow joints.

These conditions arise because with rheumatoid arthritis the immune system turns against the body and attacks the joints and organs. In some cases a person develops a single bout with the disease, which then disappears and never returns (monocyclic rheumatoid arthritis). Other times the patient cycles between periods of pain and periods of normal function (polycyclic). However, in most cases a diagnosis of rheumatoid arthritis means chronic pain—and pain management.

The diagnosis of rheumatoid arthritis can be confirmed in

about 80 percent of cases by a blood test for antibodies linked to the disease. Another test, measuring the rate of sedimentation of elements in the blood, can indicate inflammation in the joints. X rays can also confirm damage to the cartilage and bone.

The cause of rheumatoid arthritis is not fully understood. Some cases appear to be caused by a hereditary factor, but others may follow a viral infection.

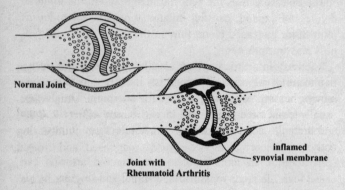

Normal Joint

Joint with Rheumatoid Arthritis

inflamed synovial membrane

Juvenile Rheumatoid Arthritis

Juvenile rheumatoid arthritis resembles rheumatoid arthritis, except that it occurs in children and teenagers. There are several types of juvenile rheumatoid arthritis:

- **Pauciarticular juvenile rheumatoid arthritis:** A type of arthritis that affects four or fewer joints, typically the large joints. About 30 to 40 percent of children with juvenile arthritis suffer from this type.
- **Polyarticular juvenile rheumatoid arthritis:** A condition that affects five or more joints, typically the small joints of the fingers and hands. This type can also settle in the weight-bearing joints. About half of the children with juvenile arthritis have this type.

- **Systemic juvenile rheumatoid arthritis:** A type of arthritis that affects the entire body, often including the internal organs in addition to the joints. A high fever and rash may accompany the joint inflammation. This is the least common type of juvenile arthritis.

Heredity appears to play some role in the development of juvenile arthritis, though the exact cause has not been determined.

Systemic Lupus Erythematosus

Arthritis is one of several symptoms of systemic lupus erythematosus, usually referred to simply as lupus. When someone develops lupus, his or her autoimmune system destroys healthy connective tissue, including the skin, joints, and internal organs. The condition, which afflicts 250,000 Americans—about 90 percent women in their childbearing years—is more manageable when diagnosed and treated early.

Though the symptoms may be present in varying degrees, common warning signs include the following:

- A rash resembling a butterfly over the bridge of the nose and cheeks
- Fever
- Fatigue
- Rapid hair loss
- Raynaud's phenomenon, a condition in which the fingers turn blue and white when exposed to cold
- Sensitivity to direct sunlight
- Mouth ulcers
- Proteinuria, or the loss of excessive amounts of protein in the urine
- Pleuritis, inflammation of the lining of the lungs
- Pericarditis, inflammation of the sac enclosing the heart

- Anemia and/or low white blood cell counts
- Kidney damage

As part of the disease many patients with lupus also develop arthritis. In such cases the disease strikes the synovial membrane of the joints, especially the wrists, knuckles, knees, and lower body. (The spine is usually not affected.) Typically the joints do not swell, but they do feel tender or painful when moved.

The cause of lupus remains unknown, though some experts suspect that heredity plays a role. The disease can be diagnosed using blood or urine analysis, X rays, and electrocardiograms.

Ankylosing Spondylitis

Ankylosing spondylitis is a type of arthritis that primarily damages the spine and sacroiliac joints, though it can also affect the shoulders, knees, ankles, heart, and lungs. In the early stages of the disease inflammatory cells invade the part of the joint where the tendons and ligaments attach to the bones. In response to the inflammation a bony ridge develops between the joints, causing them to fuse together. As the disease progresses, the spine gradually fuses together, ultimately resulting in partial or total loss of spine flexibility. The disease afflicts about 2.5 million Americans, mostly young men.

The disease is often misdiagnosed in its early stages as simple backache. The most common warning sign is a severe stiffness or loss of flexibility in the spine, which may be accompanied by fatigue and weight loss. Ankylosing spondylitis usually strikes the lower back first, then slowly moves up the spine.

In the later stages of the disease the patient's spine is frozen, usually not in an erect, upright posture but in a hunched-over position. The person often shuffles his feet because his stride has been shortened owing to the fusion of the joints in the lower back, which blocks the legs from moving through their full range of motion.

Doctors suspect that heredity plays an important role in the development of ankylosing spondylitis, and they have identified a genetic marker, HLA-B27, which is shared by most people with the disease. For some reason that is not fully understood, the disease sometimes occurs in predisposed people after they have contracted a urinary-tract or bowel infection. The diagnosis of the disease is often based on X rays, which detect evidence of spinal fusion.

Gout

Gout is a relatively common type of arthritis caused by the buildup of uric acid, a by-product of the metabolism of purines, which are made by the body and consumed in foods. During a "gout attack" the uric acid forms tiny crystals of sodium urate, which collect in a joint (often the big toe), causing inflammation and severe pain. Uric acid crystals can also be deposited in the kidneys to form kidney stones. The disease affects about one million Americans, mostly men over age forty.

Gout has long been referred to as the rich man's disease, because in the past it afflicted portly, well-to-do men who consumed a regular diet of red meat and wine. This stereotype may not be too far from the mark, since meats (especially organ meats) contain high levels of purines, and alcohol interferes with the ability of the kidneys to excrete uric acid.

Gout doesn't develop overnight. In some cases uric acid crystals may build up for years or decades before an attack. In more than half of all cases of gout, the first attack afflicts the first joint of the big toe, though it can also strike the heel, ankle, or instep. (Researchers suspect that gout appears in the extremities because uric acid forms crystals at lower temperatures, and the temperature is somewhat lower in the toes and lower extremities than at the body's core.) Often the acute pain first strikes in the middle of the night, especially after an evening of indulging in excess food and alcohol. Fever and chills may accompany the pain.

About half of all gout sufferers have a second attack within one year, and three fourths will have a recurrence within four to five years. But chronic gout is rare, since the condition can be controlled by diet and drug therapy to lower uric acid levels. Some people develop elevated uric acid levels and gout as a side effect of another disorder, such as kidney disease, which can inhibit uric acid excretion. Low-dose aspirin therapy and some diuretic high-blood-pressure treatments can also cause gout.

Doctors can confirm the diagnosis of gout by testing the uric acid levels in the blood, or by withdrawing a sample of joint fluid to look for evidence of crystals. The vast majority of gout sufferers contract the disease due to a combination of environmental factors, especially diet, but about 10 percent have a genetic predisposition to develop the disease.

Men are more susceptible to gout because uric acid levels tend to increase in males at puberty. Women tend to develop gout much later in life (usually in their sixties or later) because uric acid levels increase after menopause, when estrogen levels drop.

Pseudogout refers to a separate arthritic condition, similar to gout except that it involves the formation of calcium pyrophosphate dihydrate (CPPD) crystals in the joints. Pseudogout tends to affect the knees, wrists, and ankles most often.

Other Types of Arthritis

As mentioned earlier, more than one hundred different diseases cause pain of the joints, muscles, and bones. In addition to the more common types listed above, the following list includes other common types of arthritis and arthritislike conditions:

- *Bursitis:* A disorder causing inflammation of the bursae, small sacs containing joint-lubricating fluid, which help prevent friction inside the joint. Common locations for bursitis include the shoulders, hips, elbows, and knees.
- *Carpal tunnel syndrome:* A disorder of the wrist caused by pressure on the median nerve at the wrist. The condition, which is common in people in jobs with repetitive hand-wrist movement, can produce pain and numbness in the hand and forearm. When the wrist becomes swollen and inflamed, the nerve is compressed, causing the pain.
- *Fibromyalgia (fibrositis):* A condition that causes pain and stiffness to the soft tissue—the muscles, tendons, ligaments, and bursae—supporting the bones and joints. Other symptoms include fatigue and sleep disturbance. It usually afflicts women of childbearing age.
- *Infectious arthritis:* This type of arthritis is caused by a bacterium, virus, or fungus growing within the joint and causing inflammation. People with compromised health or early signs of joint disease are more likely to develop the problem. It can be treated with antibiotics, physical therapy, and sometimes drainage of the infected joint.
- *Lyme disease:* This infectious illness is caused by a bacterium that is spread by the bite of a tiny deer tick. The illness usually shows up as a bull's-eye rash, fever, headache, stiff neck, arthritis, and heart problems. Antibiotics can be used to treat the illness.
- *Raynaud's phenomenon:* A circulatory disorder that often accompanies other rheumatic diseases, including rheumatoid arthritis. Raynaud's phenomenon produces spasms in the blood vessels of the fingers and toes, causing them to change color—first white, then blue, and

finally red. The change usually occurs after exposure to cold or emotional stress. The condition may also involve numbness in the fingers and toes.

- *Reiter's syndrome:* This is a relatively common disease, especially in young men who have recently experienced a colon or urinary-tract infection. The disease is characterized by skin rashes, arthritis, and eye inflammation. There appears to be an inherited tendency toward the disease.
- *Scleroderma (systemic sclerosis):* An autoimmune disease that affects the blood vessels and connective tissue. Scar tissue can develop, causing a hardening of the skin,

---

PUTTING ARTHRITIS TO THE TEST

Laboratory tests can be very helpful in correct diagnosis of arthritis. Following is a rundown of a few of the most common tests:

- *Complete blood count (CBC):* This test measures the number of red and white cells in the blood. A low red blood count can indicate anemia, a common complication of rheumatoid arthritis and inflammatory disease. A low white blood count suggests the presence of infection, which may suggest infectious arthritis.
- *Erythrocyte sedimentation rate (ESR):* This test measures how fast the red blood cells clump together and settle at the bottom of a test tube of whole blood. The sedimentation rate can measure the amount of inflammation present.
- *Uric acid:* Measuring the amount of uric acid in the blood can be helpful in the diagnosis of gout. High levels of uric acid do not necessarily prove the presence of gout, but it can be an important warning sign of the disease.

as well as of the internal organs. The cause of the illness is unknown, though it appears to follow exposure to certain toxins and as a complication of organ transplants. The five-year survival rate is 60 to 70 percent.

Finding a Physician

Before launching into a self-care program, visit a doctor to confirm the diagnosis of arthritis and to rule out more serious copycat conditions. There are a number of types of medical doctors who treat arthritis:

Rheumatologists: These are doctors of internal medi-

- *Rheumatoid factor (RF, Latex):* This test looks for the antibody common to sufferers of rheumatoid arthritis. In the early stages of the disease most people will not test positive for the antibodies, but within two years 80 to 85 percent of the people with rheumatoid arthritis will test positive for the antibody.
- *Antinuclear antibody (ANA):* This test detects the presence of abnormal antibodies that attack the cell nuclei. These antibodies are usually present in people with lupus, but they may also show up in sufferers of rheumatoid arthritis and several other less common forms of the disease. The antibodies also show up in a small number of people who do not have arthritis.
- *Genetic testing:* People with ankylosing spondylitis and several other less common types of arthritis typically share a gene known as HLA-B27. Genetic testing can indicate a predisposition to this type of arthritis.
- *Synovial fluid analysis:* An analysis of the synovial fluid withdrawn from the joint can distinguish inflammatory from noninflammatory forms of arthritis. It can also be used to diagnose gout and pseudogout.

cine who have two additional years of specialized training in the treatment of arthritis and related rheumatic diseases. Rheumatologists are knowledgeable about virtually all arthritis treatments, including experimental approaches. To find a rheumatologist, ask for a referral from your current doctor or from a local medical society, the Arthritis Foundation, or the American College of Rheumatology (see ''Resources'' in Chapter 12). You might also look in the Yellow Pages of the telephone directory under ''Physicians'' and ''Rheumatology.''

Orthopedists: These doctors have at least five years of post–medical school training in diseases and injuries of the bones and joints. Orthopedists often perform joint surgery to improve joint function, but they also give nonsurgical advice on exercise, drug treatment, and pain-management techniques. (Always solicit a second opinion before opting for surgery.) To find a qualified orthopedist, ask for a referral from your physician or a local medical society. Another option would be to call the Department of Orthopedic Surgery at a hospital near you and ask for a recommendations.

Internists: These doctors of internal medicine treat patients with arthritis, but they treat other illnesses as well. Many internists will refer patients with severe arthritis to rheumatologists for specialized care. To find an internist, ask the local medical society for a referral or check in the Yellow Pages of the telephone directory under ''Physicians'' and ''Internal Medicine.''

General Practitioners: These doctors treat ''the whole patient,'' rather than specializing in the treatment of arthritis. While a general practitioner may be able to help treat mild cases of arthritis, most work in conjunction with a rheumatologist or other specialist for chronic or severe cases. To find a general practitioner, ask friends and associates for referrals, or check in the Yellow Pages of the telephone directory under "Physicians" and "General Practitioners" or "Family Practice."

As with any health care provider, if you aren't satisfied with the treatment you receive, or if you don't feel comfortable with the patient-practitioner relationship, keep looking for a practitioner better able to meet your needs. Many arthritis sufferers try several physicians before finding one who satisfies their long-term needs.

CHAPTER TWO

What You Need to Know About Conventional Treatments

When dealing with common types of arthritis most medical doctors do nothing to combat the disease. Instead they try to manage the symptoms of arthritis, often by prescribing drugs to ease the pain and reduce the inflammation. Many of these drugs work reasonably well for some patients, but often not without significant negative effects. For example a study done at a major teaching hospital in Boston showed that as many as 36 percent of patients had complications and negative side effects in response to conventional medical treatment.

The most common drugs used in the treatment of arthritis are aspirin and other nonsteroidal antiinflammatory drugs, corticosteroids, and disease-modifying drugs. In cases of advanced arthritis, when a joint has become deformed and drug therapy fails, a doctor may suggest surgery as a final option.

Aspirin and NSAIDs

Almost everyone with arthritis has sought relief from nonsteroidal antiinflammatory drugs (NSAIDs), a category of medications that includes aspirin. These drugs are available in both prescription and nonprescription formulas and can be very effective in controlling inflammation and pain—at least until a patient can no longer tolerate their negative side effects. For example at least one out of every five people taking therapeutic levels of NSAIDs develops stomach ulcers (some doctors prescribe ulcer-fighting drugs to counteract the stomach irritation caused by the NSAIDs).

NSAIDs ease the pain and inflammation of arthritis by inhibiting the formation of an enzyme that helps the body produce prostaglandins (chemicals that trigger inflammation). By cutting back on prostaglandin levels, NSAIDs can reduce the redness, warmth, pain, and swelling associated with joint inflammation.

Of course there's a catch: NSAIDs can exacerbate joint deterioration by inhibiting the body's ability to repair cartilage in the joints. In many cases high levels of NSAIDs used to control arthritis pain and inflammation can actually make the condition worse. The higher the dose and the longer the drugs are used, the greater the risk of additional joint damage, according to research published in the *Journal of Rheumatology*. Despite this devastating side effect, NSAIDs remain the first line of defense prescribed by conventional physicians, though many arthritis sufferers are not aware of their harmful effects.

Aspirin

The old-standby aspirin remains the drug of choice for most arthritis sufferers because it's cheap, widely available, and as effective as many other drugs at reducing inflammation. It has been estimated that fully half of the 22 billion aspirin tablets consumed each year in the United States are taken by people with arthritis.

For aspirin to reduce symptoms of arthritis, it must be taken in high doses—often twelve to twenty tablets a day, depending on a person's size and weight. People taking megadoses of aspirin should be monitored by a physician, who can test the aspirin (salicylate) levels in the blood using a simple blood test.

It can be tricky to keep the level high enough to be effective but low enough to avoid overdose. Aspirin overdose first shows up in most people as tinnitus (ringing in the ears). Other side effects of both aspirin and other NSAIDs include

- Ulcers and damage to the stomach lining
- Bleeding
- Fluid retention
- Decreased kidney function

Because of the side effects, aspirin and other NSAIDs should be avoided by people with kidney problems, heart disease, or cirrhosis of the liver. In addition they should be avoided by people taking blood-thinning drugs, diuretics, and other medications for diabetes and heart disease.

If you take aspirin, check the strength of the aspirin you're taking to assess your total dose. Regular aspirin has 325 milligrams of active ingredient, compared with 500 milligrams for "extra strength," "arthritis strength," or "maximum strength" tablets. Check the price; in most cases you pay more than twice as much for the extra-strength product, even though it contains less than twice as much active ingredient. High-dose formulas (800 mg or 975 mg) are available by prescription.

WARNING: Though arthritis primarily affects older people, children and adolescents with arthritis should avoid taking aspirin. The drug has been linked to Reye's syndrome, a potentially fatal disease that strikes children who take aspirin when recovering from a viral infection, such as chicken pox.

Other NSAIDs

Nonaspirin NSAIDs share many of aspirin's negative side effects (see page 18), but they offer one major advantage: They are more potent, so you need fewer tablets to reach a therapeutic level. For example, 100 milligrams of one NSAID may be the equivalent of 1,000 milligrams of aspirin. On the downside, other NSAIDs tend to be considerably more expensive than aspirin.

Some NSAIDs, such as ibuprofen, are available in both prescription and nonprescription versions. The only difference between the two is strength: The over-the-counter version has 200 milligrams of ibuprofen per tablet, compared with 400, 600, or 800 milligrams, depending on the strength of the prescription.

THREE WAYS TO PROTECT YOUR STOMACH

1. **Dilute.** Drink a glass of water or milk when you take aspirin or another NSAID. Avoid alcoholic beverages, which can further irritate or damage the stomach lining.
2. **Buffer.** Eat something when you take your medication to avoid high concentrations of aspirin or another NSAID against the stomach lining. Of course eating a four-course dinner will slow the absorption of the drug into your bloodstream if you're looking for immediate pain relief. However, if you're taking the medication to keep a constant therapeutic level of drug in your body, then the meal will protect your stomach without interfering with the medication in your bloodstream.
3. **Counteract.** If necessary, consider taking an antiulcer or stomach-soothing drug for protection. Talk to your doctor about the possibility of taking Maalox, Mylanta, Tagamet, or Cytotec.

COMMON NONASPIRIN NSAIDS

Every person responds differently to NSAIDs. If you want to use NSAIDs in your arthritis treatment, you and your doctor may have to go through a trial-and-error process to find a drug that works for you without causing unpleasant or intolerable side effects.

ACTIVE INGREDIENT	BRAND NAMES
Diclofenac sodium	Voltaren
Diflunisal	Dolobid
Fenoprofen	Nalfon
Flurbiprofen	Ansaid
Ibuprofen*	Motrin, Advil, Nuprin
Indomethacin	Indocin
Ketoprofen*	Orudis
Meclofenamate	Meclomen
Mefenamic acid	Ponstel
Naproxen*	Anaprox, Naprosyn, Aleve
Piroxicam	Feldene
Sulindac	Clinoril
Tolmetin	Tolectin

* A nonprescription version of this drug is available.

Corticosteroids

More than fifty years ago doctors noticed that the condition of women with rheumatoid arthritis often improved during pregnancy. They examined the hormones produced during pregnancy and considered the possibility that arthritis responded to cortisol, a hormone produced by the outer part of the adrenal gland. When injections of this corticosteroid were administered to arthritis patients as part of an experiment, they were given new life: Those who had been crippled by the disease for years were able suddenly to walk, move about, and even dance again.

As the researchers discovered, corticosteroids quickly reduce inflammation. But they soon realized that corticosteroids were not the miracle drugs they had been looking for, because of the dangerous side effects. In the body corticosteroids block the production of substances that trigger allergic and inflammatory reactions; this helped offer short-term relief from swelling, but left the people on the drug more susceptible to infection and disease. Other negative side effects include increased appetite and weight gain, water and salt retention, high blood pressure, diabetes, thin skin, osteoporosis, cataracts, acne, muscle weakness, stomach ulcers, mental disorders, and adrenal suppression.

Pharmaceutical companies have since developed synthetic versions of the hormone, which are still used, though in a more limited way. About thirty corticosteroids have been developed and approved as safe and effective by the U.S. Food and Drug Administration, provided they are used as directed. They are primarily used when arthritis fails to respond to other medications; the drugs can be taken orally or injected into the joints to provide temporary relief (from a few days to a few months).

Commonly used corticosteroids include cortisone (Cortone), dexamethasone (Decadrol, Decadron), hydrocortisone or cortisol (Cortef, Hydrocortone), methylprednisolone (Niscort, Hydeltrasol, Medrol), prednisone (Deltasone), and prednisolone (Delta-Cortef).

Disease-Modifying Drugs

Rheumatoid arthritis can also be treated by a category of drugs referred to as disease-modifying (they stop the disease process), slow-acting (they can take months to become effective), or remittive (in some cases they push the disease into remission). No matter what they're called, these drugs can have a powerful effect in changing the progress of the disease.

Gold

Gold has been used in the treatment of arthritis for more than seventy years. The initial discovery was an accident: Testing a theory that metals could be used to treat infections, a French physician injected gold salts into some of his tuberculosis patients, who also had arthritis. The TB failed to improve, but the arthritis symptoms began to fade. Gold has been used to treat rheumatoid arthritis ever since.

No one knows exactly how the gold works in the body, but it seems to interfere with the functions of white blood cells that cause joint damage. Gold can't reverse existing joint deformities, though in some patients it does slow or halt additional damage.

Gold capsules taken orally have recently begun to replace injections. The pills (auranofin [Ridaura]) must be taken twice a day; gold injections must be done about once a week during the first few months. The gold compound is injected into a muscle in the buttock, and the amount is increased gradually.

Any patient taking gold treatments must be monitored for toxic side effects, including kidney and liver damage and bone marrow suppression. Skin rashes and sores in the mouth are also common. The oral treatments tend to cause fewer side effects, diarrhea being the most common. Because of the side effects, gold treatment is usually used only in cases when the arthritis fails to respond to other medications.

Gold treatments don't work on everyone. Roughly six out of ten patients respond very well to the treatment, two or three get some relief, and one or two do not experience any improvement.

Immunosuppressive Drugs

In certain cases potent immunosuppressive drugs are used to control rheumatoid arthritis and other immune-system forms of the disease. As the name implies, immunosuppressive drugs suppress the immune system by slowing cell division and making the entire immune system sluggish. Remember, in rheumatoid arthritis the body's immune system attacks the joints, so slowing the system helps slow the progression of the disease.

Of course these drugs have significant side effects. By changing the immune system, the body is less capable of fighting infection and injury. The major immunosuppressive drugs include azathioprine (Imuran), chlorambucil (Leukeran), cyclophosphamide (Cytoxan), methotrexate, and hydroxychloroquine (Plaquenil). A study published in the *New England Journal of Medicine* in July 1995 found that combination therapy—using two immunosuppressive drugs simultaneously—resulted in greater improvement than using either drug alone.

QUESTIONS TO ASK YOUR DOCTOR BEFORE TAKING ANY DRUG

Before filling a prescription for an arthritis medication—or any other drug for that matter—be sure to ask your doctor or pharmacist a number of questions:

- How soon will this medication begin to work?
- What results should I expect?
- What are the possible side effects?
- Should I report the side effects to you or stop taking the drug?
- Should I take the medication with a meal or on an empty stomach?
- Are there any foods I should avoid when taking this drug?
- Can I consume alcohol when taking this drug?
- Could this drug interact with any other prescription drugs I am currently taking? With any over-the-counter drugs? With any vitamin or mineral supplements?
- How long should I expect to take this drug?
- Can I automatically renew the prescription if necessary?
- If I feel better, should I take less of the drug?
- Is this drug habit-forming?
- Is there a generic form of the drug, or should I take it as written?

In addition be sure to read the prescription before leaving the doctor's office, making sure you understand the correct spelling of the drug name. When you pick up the filled prescription from the pharmacist, double-check the drug name written on the prescription with the drug name typed on the drug bottle.

Treatment of Gout

Most cases of gout can be managed by diet alone, but a number of drugs can be effective in managing gout attacks. In most cases of chronic gout a doctor will take urine samples twenty-four hours apart and assess the level of uric acid in the samples to find out whether the problem is caused by the overproduction or underexcretion of uric acid. A doctor may also prescribe one of the following drugs:

Colchicine

This drug is often used when a doctor isn't certain about the diagnosis of gout. Colchicine lowers the acidity of the joints, stopping the inflammation and dissolving the uric acid crystals. If the problem is gout, the drug brings almost instant relief. If it isn't gout, the drug offers no relief.

The drug has significant side effects, including abdominal cramps, vomiting, nausea, and diarrhea. The higher the dose, the greater the likelihood of other, more severe side effects, such as hair loss, bone marrow suppression, liver damage, and bloody diarrhea caused by colon inflammation. Considering the unpleasant possible side effects, controlling the disease through diet should seem like an appealing alternative.

Allopurinol

This drug is usually prescribed for someone who produces too much uric acid. Allopurinol inhibits the formation of uric acid by interfering with the activity of the enzyme responsible for the metabolism of purines into uric acid. The most common side effect from allopurinol is a skin rash, which can be severe. Other side effects include headache, dizziness, fatigue, and liver damage.

Sulfinpyrazone

This drug is usually prescribed for someone who overproduces uric acid. Sulfinpyrazone increases the body's excretion of uric acid, which increases the possibility of developing kidney stones. People with kidney problems should not take sulfinpyrazone. Other possible side effects include nausea, vomiting, abdominal cramping, headache, and liver damage.

Surgery

In advanced cases of arthritis, reconstructive surgery is sometimes necessary to restore joint function. During most procedures the joint is removed and replaced with an implant made of synthetic materials, usually metal alloys in the large joints and polymers in the small joints. New implants are often coated with a material containing calcium phosphate, which can allow the implant to interact with and "cement" to the bone.

More than one million people have had joint replacements, most often hip and knee replacements. During "implant resection arthroplasty," the official name for implant joint surgery, the doctor removes the damaged cartilage and part of the bone and cements the implant onto the bone. The muscles, tendons, and ligaments are then reattached.

As with any surgical procedure, joint replacement has some risk, primarily the risk of the anesthesia during the surgery and the risk of infection after surgery. But these risks are relatively small; for example less than one percent of all hip replacements become infected. There is also some risk that the implant will become loosened, dislocated, worn down, or broken. In most cases these mechanical problems can be repaired without additional surgery.

Another type of joint surgery involves arthroscopy, in

which the joint is viewed by a light inserted into the tissue through a small incision. The damaged cartilage is then surgically corrected, but without opening up the entire joint. The recovery time for arthroscopic surgery is typically much shorter than that for joint replacement, but the procedure is appropriate only in relatively mild cases of osteoarthritis, because in severe cases the cartilage is either gone or too severely damaged to repair.

Common Drugs Used for Arthritis

DRUG CATEGORY	TYPES OF ARTHRITIS FOR WHICH THE DRUG IS COMMONLY USED	HOW IT WORKS	COMMON SIDE EFFECTS
Aspirin	Most types, except gout	Limits the production of substances that cause pain, swelling, warmth, and redness	Gastrointestinal upset Bleeding Fluid retention Liver inflammation Ringing in ears
Other NSAIDs	All types of arthritis	Limits the production of substances that cause pain, swelling, warmth, and redness	Stomach pain Gastrointestinal upset Bleeding Fluid retention Kidney damage
Corticosteroids	Osteoarthritis Rheumatoid	Blocks release of	Increased appetite

DRUG CATEGORY	TYPES OF ARTHRITIS FOR WHICH THE DRUG IS COMMONLY USED	HOW IT WORKS	COMMON SIDE EFFECTS
	arthritis Lupus Scleroderma	inflammatory agents and suppresses white blood cells to rapidly reduce inflammation	Weight gain Fat in chest, face, and upper back Water retention High blood pressure Osteoporosis Thinning skin Cataracts Acne Muscle weakness Susceptibility to infection Ulcers Depression
Disease-modifying Drugs (including gold)	Rheumatoid arthritis Lupus Scleroderma	Most of these drugs alter the immune function	Varies by drug, but typically: Skin rash Mouth sores Kidney damage Diarrhea Stomach upset Liver damage Nausea

Drug Category	Types of Arthritis for Which the Drug Is Commonly Used	How It Works	Common Side Effects
			Loss of appetite
Immunosuppressive Drugs	Rheumatoid arthritis Lupus	Blocks cell growth, suppresses white blood cells, some by binding with cell DNA	Varies by drug, but typically: Gastrointestinal upset Heartburn Susceptibility to infection Bleeding Bruising Hair loss Kidney damage

CHAPTER THREE

Food as Medicine: Controlling Arthritis Through Diet

Food isn't just food; it is medicine for the body. A well-balanced, nutritious diet can help ward off arthritis pain and joint degeneration, just as a diet high in processed foods, animal fat, and certain trigger foods can make arthritis symptoms noticeably worse. And don't forget that eating a wholesome diet also helps prevent heart disease, diabetes, certain types of cancer, and a multitude of diseases associated with being overweight.

First, a Word About Weight

No matter what type of arthritis you have, the more extra weight you carry around, the greater the chances your joints will hurt. Think about it: If you had an injured knee, you wouldn't want to lug around a thirty-pound bag of gravel all day, would you? There's no difference to your knees between thirty pounds of fat and thirty pounds of gravel. Losing any excess weight will improve your overall health and make the weight-bearing joints feel less stressed.

ARE YOU OVERWEIGHT?

Most of us can tell if we're overweight by looking in a mirror, but the following table provides more specific target weights:

Healthy Weight Ranges for Men and Women

HEIGHT (without shoes)	WEIGHT IN POUNDS (without clothes)
4' 10"	91–119
4' 11"	94–124
5' 0"	97–128
5' 1"	101–132
5' 2"	104–137
5' 3"	107–141
5' 4"	111–146
5' 5"	114–150
5' 6"	118–155
5' 7"	121–160
5' 8"	125–164
5' 9"	129–169
5' 10"	132–174
5' 11"	136–179
6' 0"	140–184
6' 1"	144–189
6' 2"	148–195
6' 3"	152–200
6' 4"	156–205
6' 5"	160–211
6' 6"	164–216

Source: U.S. Dietary Guidelines for Americans, 1995.

Weight problems tend to be more common for people with osteoarthritis than those with rheumatoid arthritis. And every additional pound makes use of the joints—particularly the knee and hip joints—more painful, which tempts sedentary folks to sit down, relax, and gain additional weight rather than exercise and shed those unwanted pounds.

If you are overweight and lose weight, regardless of the weight-reduction diet you follow, you will feel better and almost certainly experience some pain relief. One of your first goals in designing a diet to manage your arthritis pain should be to reach and maintain a normal body weight if you are overweight.

Unfortunately there are no shortcuts to weight reduction. The only way to lose weight is to burn more calories than you consume. It is best to design a weight-loss plan that involves the loss of no more than two pounds per week. Remember, one pound of fat contains 3,500 calories.

The number of calories any individual needs depends on age, sex, and lifestyle. The following calorie-intake tables may be helpful in coming up with a diet plan that meets your needs:

Men

Age 18–35	Inactive	2,500 calories/day
	Active	3,000 calories/day
	Very active	3,500 calories/day
Age 36–70	Inactive	2,400 calories/day
	Active	2,800 calories/day
	Very active	3,400 calories/day

Women

Age 18–55	Inactive	1,900 calories/day
	Active	2,100 calories/day
	Very active	2,500 calories/day
Age 56–70	Inactive	1,700 calories/day
	Active	2,000 calories/day
	Very active	2,100 calories/day

In order to lose weight, you would have to consume fewer calories than indicated in the table. But don't count calories without regard to their source. The key to good nutrition is balance. Eat a variety of whole foods from the basic food groups while limiting your intake of fats. Losing weight is never easy, but it can make an important difference in your arthritis pain—as well as your overall health.

Food and Osteoarthritis

Osteoarthritis involves the gradual degeneration of the cartilage and joint tissue. Diet and nutrition can help prevent—and sometimes reverse—osteoarthritis by nourishing the joints and supporting the body's efforts to heal itself.

If you suffer from osteoarthritis, you may be able to manage the disease by carefully monitoring your diet.

- **Eat plenty of fruits and vegetables.** Plant foods contain antioxidants, compounds that protect the body against cellular damage caused by free radicals and pro-oxidants. Free radicals, which are created during metabolism, cause chronic degenerative diseases, including osteoarthritis. Free radicals also come from cigarette smoking, sunlight, X rays, pesticides, formaldehyde, and aromatic hydrocarbons, among other environmental sources. Plant foods rich in antioxidants, such as beta-carotenes, flavonoids, selenium, zinc, and vitamins C and E, help wipe out or neutralize free radicals.

- **Go for the garlic.** Sulfur-containing foods—garlic, onions, Brussels sprouts, and cabbage—help control arthritis symptoms. Research shows that the fingernails of people with arthritis have significantly less sulfur than the fingernails of healthy people. To avoid the bad-breath dilemma, encourage your spouse or partner to share in your sulfur-rich foods, or take odorless garlic supplements.

- **Pass on certain veggies.** Eliminating vegetables from the nightshade family—tomatoes, potatoes, eggplants, and peppers—can promote cartilage repair. The nightshade vegetables contain high levels of alkaloids, which may trigger problems in susceptible people. The theory is that alkaloids remove calcium from the bones and deposit it in the joints, causing calcification, inflammation, and pain. An estimated 70 percent of arthritis sufferers who avoid nightshade-family vegetables report some relief from joint pain.

- **Skip the aspartame.** The artificial sweetener aspartame doesn't cause arthritis, but it has been reported to cause joint pain in people who consume moderate amounts of it. If your joints hurt, pass on the aspartame and see if it helps ease the pain.

Food and Rheumatoid Arthritis

Rheumatoid arthritis is caused by a number of factors, including diet and food allergies. Even conservative physicians are starting to consider the possibility of a link between diet and rheumatoid arthritis. Remember, mainstream cardiologists once scoffed at the idea that diet could affect heart disease or cancer, but today they accept the importance of nutrition in controlling disease.

Almost any food can aggravate rheumatoid arthritis, but the most common food allergens are corn, wheat products, milk and dairy products, beef, pork, alcohol, nuts, and nightshade vegetables (see the previous section, ''Food and Osteoarthritis''). Food additives, dyes, and preservatives can also cause problems.

A reaction toward a food can happen within minutes or up to several hours after eating the food, and symptoms vary enormously. They can include diarrhea, vomiting, runny nose, rashes, hives, itching, and swelling in the lips, mouth, or throat. At the most extreme, food allergies can cause anaphylactic shock, in which the immune, respiratory, and circulatory systems react simultaneously, sometimes causing coma or death.

No single food allergen triggers arthritis pain in all people, so it's up to you to work through an elimination diet to identify an allergy if you have one. It can be a long and tedious process to identify a food allergy. (The task is often made more difficult because many people are allergic to more than one food.)

There are two ways of conducting an elimination diet. You can either eliminate the one food suspected of causing problems, then wait several days to see if your symptoms subside, or you can attempt to systematically test all the foods in your diet. To conduct a full-diet test, you should fast for two or three days (if your doctor approves), then introduce one new food every second day. If you notice an increase in joint pain or swelling within two to forty-eight hours, omit this food from your diet for a week, then try introducing it again. If symptoms return again, cut this food from your diet. The process is time-consuming because it can take long periods to identify the offending foods.

An article published in 1988 in *Annals of the Rheumatic Diseases* concluded that ''a high proportion of patients improved on dietary manipulations and that there was marked individual variation in response to the elimination of different dietary items.'' In other words there is no simple solution, but if you work at it, you may be able to find considerable relief by changing your diet.

Some experts believe food allergies are rare, occurring in only 5 to 10 percent of people with arthritis, but that others may have a food sensitivity or intolerance that is strong enough to trigger a reaction even if the body does not mount an all-out allergic reaction.

In addition to identifying any food allergies, you can help to deal with rheumatoid arthritis by following these dietary guidelines:

- **Cut back on saturated fats.** Fatty acids can decrease— or increase—joint inflammation, depending on the type of oil you consume. Saturated fats are animal fats that are solid or semisolid at room temperatures; they can make arthritis pain worse. On the other hand fish oils containing omega-3 fatty acids may help relieve inflammation and arthritis pain. Fish high in omega-3 acids include anchovies, Atlantic and pink salmon, lake trout, mackerel, herring, and bluefish.
- **Eat plenty of fruits and vegetables.** (See the previous section ''Food and Osteoarthritis.'')
- **Please pass the flavonoids.** Flavonoids are the pigments that give fruits and flowers their color. In the body flavonoids have antiinflammatory, antiallergic, and antiviral properties, in addition to scavenging the body for harmful oxidants and free radicals. The flavonoids found in blueberries, cherries, grapes, and blackberries support the joint structures and collagen formation, so head for the fruit stand and start snacking.

FLAVONOID-RICH FOODS

Fruits:

Apples	Grapes (red)
Apricots	Hawthorn berries
Blueberries	Peaches
Cherries	Plums
Cowberries	Raspberries
Cranberries	Strawberries
Currants (black)	

Other:

Parsley	Sage
Rhubarb	Wine (red)

Food and Gout

Even the most conservative physicians recognize the link between diet and gout. The consumption of purines—substances found in certain foods, including organ meats and sardines—can raise levels of uric acid in the bloodstream, triggering a gout attack. Alcohol can also bring on an attack, because alcohol interferes with the body's ability to metabolize purines.

If you suffer from gout, you can help control outbreaks by sticking to the following dietary guidelines:

- **Just say no to alcohol.** Alcohol increases levels of gout-causing uric acid in the bloodstream by impairing the kidneys' ability to excrete the substance. As a result drinking alcohol can trigger a gout attack.
- **Pass up the purines.** Cutting purine-containing foods from your diet is one of the best ways to control out-

breaks of gout. That means eliminating from your diet anchovies, brewer's and baker's yeast, herring, mackerel, organ meat, sardines, and shellfish.

- **Lose weight if necessary.** Trimming down to your ideal body weight lowers uric acid levels in the blood. Not surprisingly most people who suffer from gout are obese.
- **Cut back on refined carbohydrates and saturated fats.** Try to minimize your intake of refined carbohydrates (which increase the production of uric acid in the blood) and saturated fats (which decrease the secretion of uric acid in the blood).
- **Drink plenty of fluids.** Drinking at least eight 8-ounce glasses of water each day helps to dilute the urine and encourages the body to excrete excess uric acid.
- **Snack on cherries and berries.** Cherries, blueberries, and other dark red or blue berries contain high levels of flavonoid compounds called anthocyanidins and proanthocyanidins. Eating a half-pound of these berries a day helps lower uric acid levels.

TIPS ON EATING RIGHT

- **Eat a variety of foods.** The human body needs more than forty different essential nutrients. The best way to be sure you get all the nutrients you need is to eat a variety of foods from different food groups.
- **Eat foods high in fiber.** Fiber is the undigested part of the plants we eat. Fiber adds bulk to the stools and aids digestion.
- **Cook smart.** Broil, bake, grill, and poach rather than frying and using high-fat cooking methods.
- **Read food labels.** Keep an eye out for additives, preservatives, and other ingredients that might exacerbate an arthritic condition. Scrutinize labels for trigger foods if you know that you have a food allergy.
- **Drink plenty of fluids.** Drink at least eight 8-ounce glasses of water a day.
- **Eat breakfast.** The morning meal should supply one fourth of your daily nutrients, in addition to helping to control your appetite throughout the day.

RESOURCES: DIET AND NUTRITION

For information on finding a qualified nutritional counselor, contact:

The Consumer Nutrition Hotline
(sponsored by the American Dietetic Association)
(800) 366-1655
The Hotline staff can answer questions and provide free referrals to registered dietitians in your area.

You can also request referrals of certified nutritional consultants by contacting:

American Academy of Nutrition
3408 Sausalito Drive
Corona Del Mar, California 92625
(800) 290-4226

The American Association of Nutritional Consultants
880 Canarios Court, Suite 210
Chula Vista, California 91910-7810
(619) 482-8533

Publications on nutrition are available (some for a fee) from:

American Council on Science and Health
1995 Broadway, 16th Floor
New York, New York 10023-5860
(212) 362-7044

American Institute of Nutrition
9650 Rockville Pike, Suite L4500
Bethesda, Maryland 20814-3990
(301) 530-7050

Society for Nutrition Education
2001 Killebrew Drive, Suite 340
Minneapolis, Minnesota 55425-1882
(612) 854-0035

For information on food allergies, contact:

American Academy of Allergy, Asthma, and Immunology
611 East Wells Street
Milwaukee, Wisconsin 53202
(414) 272-6071

American Allergy Association
P.O. Box 7273
Menlo Park, California 94026
(415) 322-1663

Asthma and Allergy Foundation of America
1125 15th Street, NW
Suite 502
Washington, DC 20005
(202) 466-7643

The Food Allergy Network
10400 Eaton Place, Suite 107
Fairfax, Virginia 22030-2208
(800) 929-4040

CHAPTER FOUR

When More Is (Usually) Better: Vitamins and Supplements

Ideally you would get all the vitamins and minerals you need from the foods you eat. But eating an ideal diet isn't always possible, and the body isn't always as efficient as it should be at extracting nutrients from food. In fact after around age fifty the body's ability to absorb nutrients begins to drop off, increasing the possibility of nutritional deficiencies.

By taking vitamin and mineral supplements you can make up for any lapses in your nutritional intake. The federal government has established recommended dietary allowances (RDAs) for essential nutrients, using information provided by the Food and Nutrition Board of the National Academy of Sciences National Research Council. The RDAs vary with age and sex, though in an attempt to simplify matters, a single RDA is used on food labels.

Even the most conservative physicians would agree that taking supplements to meet the RDAs is not harmful, but self-diagnosing and taking megadoses of specific vitamins can be. When the body encounters large doses of water-soluble vitamins, the excess that the body can't use is simply excreted in the urine. However, fat-soluble vitamins can accumulate in the body and cause potential health problems. There is an appropriate range of vitamin intake, and as the following charts show, consuming too little or too much of some nutrients can be dangerous.

Supplements and Osteoarthritis

Changing your diet can go a long way toward easing the symptoms of osteoarthritis, but nutritional supplements may offer additional benefits.

• **Glucosamine sulfate.** As people age, their bodies produce less glucosamine sulfate, a substance found inside the joints that helps in the formation of cartilage. Without enough glucosamine, cartilage loses water and becomes a less effective cushion. Fortunately taking glucosamine supplements helps to reverse the effects of osteoarthritis.

Glucosamine is not an antiinflammatory or pain-relieving drug, but several double-blind studies have shown that glucosamine sulfate reduces swelling and pain better than nonsteroidal antiinflammatory drugs (NSAIDs). The longer glucosamine is used, the more striking the results: One study that compared glucosamine sulfate to ibuprofen found that pain decreased somewhat faster in the first two weeks among patients taking ibuprofen, but by week four the glucosamine group felt significantly better than the ibuprofen group.

Glucosamine sulfate is available at health food stores and from some physicians. The standard dose is 500 milligrams, three times a day, but follow the directions provided by your doctor or on the product label. Be sure to pick up glucosamine sulfate, rather than glucosamine hydrochloride, since the research on effectiveness has been performed on the sulfate form.

Key Fat-Soluble Vitamins

NOTE: Before taking therapeutic doses of any nutritional supplement, discuss the matter with your health care provider.

VITAMIN	ROLE IN THE BODY	ADULT RDA	SIGNS OF DEFICIENCY	FOOD SOURCES	THERAPEUTIC DOSE	SIGNS OF OVERDOSE
Vitamin A (beta-carotene)	Boosts immune system, strengthens mucous membranes, promotes bone development	5,000 IU	Night blindness, eye problems, frequent infections, diarrhea	Fish liver oil, dark green leafy vegetables, fortified milk, egg yolks, butter, pumpkin, apricots	5,000–10,000 IU	Fatigue, fluid retention, headache, vomiting
Vitamin D	Supports bone formation, necessary for	400 IU	Bone and tooth problems, rickets	Fish liver oil, fortified milk, sunshine,	100 IU	Headache, nausea, protein in urine,

	absorption of calcium, phosphorus, magnesium, and zinc	100–400 IU		salmon, herring, sardines, egg yolk	thirst, weakness, vomiting
Vitamin E	Aids tissue healing, helps form red blood cells, necessary for enzyme function	30 IU	Dry skin	Wheat germ oil, wheat germ, egg yolks, liver, nuts, whole wheat flour, green leafy vegetables, margarine, butter	Diarrhea, nausea

Key Water-Soluble Vitamins

VITAMIN	ROLE IN THE BODY	ADULT RDA	SIGNS OF DEFICIENCY	FOOD SOURCES	THERAPEUTIC DOSE	SIGNS OF OVERDOSE
Vitamin B_1 (thiamine)	Necessary for healthy heart, muscles, nerves; helps break down carbohydrates	1.5 mg	Fatigue, memory loss, depression, confusion	Brewer's yeast, kidney, liver, wheat germ, peas, peanuts, whole grains, nuts, brown rice, pork, legumes	1.5 mg	Nontoxic
Vitamin B_2 (riboflavin)	Helps break down proteins, carbohydrates, and fats; supports cell energy products;	1.3 mg (female) 1.8 mg (male)	Sensitivity to light, red eyes, dry skin, depression	Brewer's yeast, kidney, liver, milk, broccoli, Brussels sprouts, asparagus,	2 mg	Bright yellow urine

Vitamin	Function		Deficiency	Sources		Toxicity
	good for the eyes			wheat germ, almonds, cottage cheese, yogurt, eggs, tuna, salmon		
Vitamin B$_3$ (niacin)	Necessary for nervous and digestive systems and production of sex hormones; helps maintain skin	15 mg (female) 20 mg (male)	Fatigue, irritability, insomnia, blood sugar fluctuations, arthritis	Brewer's yeast, liver, poultry, fish, peanuts, eggs, milk, whole grains	18 mg	Flushed face or hands, nausea, diarrhea
Vitamin B$_5$ (pantothenic acid)	Breaks down carbohydrates and fats, supports normal growth, neces-	4–7 mg	Deficiency in other B vitamins	Liver, kidney, fish, egg yolks, cheese, brain, whole-grain cereals,	50 mg	Nontoxic

Vitamin	Role in the Body	Adult RDA	Signs of Deficiency	Food Sources	Therapeutic Dose	Signs of Overdose
	sary for production of sex hormones			cauliflower, sweet potatoes, nuts		
Vitamin B$_6$ (pyridoxine)	Helps production of red blood cells and antibodies, used in functioning of nervous and digestive systems	1.5 mg (female) 2 mg (male)	Depression, irritability	Soybeans, liver, kidney, poultry, tuna, fish, bananas, legumes, potatoes, oatmeal, wheat germ	2.5 mg	Nontoxic
Vitamin B$_{12}$ (cobalamin)	Helps in production of red blood cells,	3 mcg	Anemia, irritability, loss of coordination	Liver, oysters, poultry, fish, clams, eggs,	5–250 mcg	Nontoxic

Name	Function		Deficiency	Sources		Toxicity
	helps body use folic acid, supports nervous system			dairy products		
Biotin	Helps metabolize fatty acids, carbohydrates, and protein; helps maintain bone marrow, nerves, skin, and hair	100–200 mcg	High cholesterol, skin problems, muscle cramps	Liver, kidney, egg yolk, milk, yeast, whole grains, cauliflower, nuts, legumes	200 mcg	Nontoxic
Folic Acid	Necessary for growth and reproduction, used in production of red	400 mcg	Anemia, digestive problems, fatigue	Liver, salmon, eggs, asparagus, green leafy vegetables, sweet po-	400 mcg	Nontoxic

Vitamin	Role in the Body	Adult RDA	Signs of Deficiency	Food Sources	Therapeutic Dose	Signs of Overdose
	blood cells, supports nervous system			tatoes, beans, whole wheat		
Vitamin C	Used for growth of teeth, bones, gums, ligaments, blood vessels; important to immune system and wound healing	60 mg	Slow wound healing, bleeding gums, recurrent infections, allergies, bruise easily	Rose hips, sweet peppers, broccoli, cauliflower, kale, asparagus, spinach, tomatoes, lemons, strawberries, papayas, cantaloupe, oranges, grapefruit, mangoes	300–3,000 mg	Diarrhea, kidney stones, nausea

Key Minerals and Trace Elements

Mineral or Element	Role in the Body	Adult RDA	Signs of Deficiency	Food Sources	Therapeutic Dose	Signs of Overdose
Calcium	Helps bone and tooth formation, blood clotting, heart rhythm, cell membranes	800 mg (adults) 1,000 mg (older women) 1,200 mg (pregnant and breast-feeding women)	Muscle cramps, irritability, insomnia	Collards, turnip greens, broccoli, kale, yogurt, milk, diary products, tofu	1,200 mg	Calcium deposits, kidney stones
Magnesium	Helps blood sugar metabolism, supports DNA and RNA	325 mg (adults) 450 mg (pregnant and breast-feeding women)	Depression, muscle tension and cramps, constipation, fatigue, nervousness	Soybeans, whole grains, shellfish, salmon, liver, cashews, bananas,	400 mg	Confusion, fatigue, slow heart rate, weakness

Mineral or Element	Role in the Body	Adult RDA	Signs of Deficiency	Food Sources	Therapeutic Dose	Signs of Overdose
				potatoes, milk, green vegetables		
Chromium	Supports circulatory system, helps maintain blood sugar level	50–200 mcg	Blood sugar fluctuations, high cholesterol	Brewer's yeast, liver, cheese, legumes, whole grains, peas, molasses	200 mcg	Nontoxic
Iron	Helps produce hemoglobin, necessary for growth of children	12 mg (male) 15 mg (female)	Fatigue, anemia, intolerance of cold	Molasses, liver, eggs, fish, spinach, prunes, raisins, asparagus	18 mg	Diarrhea, vomiting, weak pulse

	Function	Dosage	Deficiency Symptoms	Food Sources	Excess Symptoms
Selenium	Helps body use vitamin E, necessary for cell membranes, supports pancreas	50 mcg	Dry scalp, skin problems	Whole grains, soybeans, tuna, seafood, pineapples, brown rice	Dental cavities, hair loss, nail loss, nervous system problems
Zinc	Supports wound healing, boosts immune system, helps digestion of carbohydrates and protein	15 mg (adults) 20 mg (pregnant and breast-feeding women)	White spots on fingernails, joint pain, slow wound healing, acne, recurrent infection	Brewer's yeast, liver, wheat germ, bran, oatmeal, carrots, sunflower seeds, spinach	Dehydration, fatigue, kidney failure, vomiting

Glucosamine has few side effects and rarely causes adverse reactions when taken with other drugs (including NSAIDs); if you experience nausea, heartburn, or other gastrointestinal upset, try taking the product with meals.

• **Cartilage extracts.** Health food stores carry a variety of products for osteoarthritis designed to improve cartilage function and formation. The cartilage extracts—often shark cartilage, sea cucumbers, and green-lipped mussels—contain molecules made up of glucosamine sulfate and sugar. Rather than using cartilage extracts, take glucosamine sulfate in its pure form, which can be more easily absorbed by the body.

• **Vitamins C and E.** Both vitamins C and E are antioxidants, which help prevent damage to cartilage in the joints among other health benefits. Vitamin C also assists in the manufacture of collagen, a protein in cartilage. Without enough vitamin C, the body stops producing collagen and the joints become compromised.

How much vitamin C should be taken by someone with osteoarthritis is open to debate. Some researchers recommend doses of 2 to 9 grams daily, arguing that any amount not needed by the body will be excreted because vitamin C is a water-soluble vitamin. Others argue that the U.S. RDA is 60 milligrams a day, and supplements should not exceed 300 to 500 milligrams a day. To decide what level of supplementation is right for you, discuss the issue with your health care provider. And of course eat plenty of foods rich in vitamin C.

Studies have also shown that vitamin E helps protect against cartilage breakdown, especially when taken in combination with vitamin C. Again, the level of supplementation is in question, anywhere from 100 IU to 600 IU a day. Before deciding how much vitamin E to take each day, talk the issue over with your physician.

• **Vitamin B$_3$ (niacin and niacinamide).** Studies have shown that vitamin B$_3$ can be helpful in treating osteoarthritis when taken at high doses. Niacinamide and niacin are both forms of vitamin B$_3$, but niacinamide appears to be better tolerated by the body. Still, vitamin B$_3$ can be toxic at high doses, so take therapeutic supplements only under a doctor's supervision. Your doctor will perform a blood test every few months to monitor your liver function to protect against overdose.

• **Boron.** Boron is necessary for the formation and maintenance of cartilage, but boron is not included in many multiple-vitamin, multiple-mineral formulas because the federal government has not established an RDA for boron. If you have osteoarthritis and your daily vitamin routine does not include boron, consider taking a supplement that provides 6 to 9 milligrams a day of the mineral.

Most dietary boron comes from fruits and vegetables. But the amount of boron in foods reflects the amount of boron in the soil where the food is grown. Studies have shown that people living in areas with low levels of environmental boron tend to have higher rates of osteoarthritis.

Studies have also shown that supplementation works. A study published in the *Journal of Nutritional Medicine* found that among people with osteoarthritis taking 6 milligrams of boron daily, more than 70 percent improved, compared with just 10 percent of the group taking a placebo.

• **Vitamin A, copper, and zinc.** To produce collagen and cartilage, the body needs an adequate supply of vitamin A, copper, and zinc. Take a multiple-vitamin, multiple-mineral supplement that includes the RDA for vitamin A, copper, and zinc. High doses should not be necessary.

Supplements and Rheumatoid Arthritis

Rheumatoid arthritis has also been shown to respond to certain types of nutrient supplementation.

• **Selenium and vitamin E.** Many people with rheumatoid arthritis have been found to have low levels of selenium, an important antioxidant that also helps slow the body's production of inflammatory agents called prostaglandins and leukotrienes. When taken with vitamin E, another antioxidant, studies have found that the supplements help ease pain and inflammation associated with rheumatoid arthritis.

In addition a recent study from Finland found that these antioxidants can help stave off the disease in the first place. The study, published in 1994 in *Annals of the Rheumatic Diseases,* found that people with low levels of vitamin E, selenium, and beta-carotene (another antioxidant) in their bloodstreams were eight times more likely than people with the highest levels to develop rheumatoid arthritis.

Most good multiple-vitamin, multiple-mineral supplements contain appropriate amounts of selenium (50–200 mcg) and vitamin E (100–400 IU). Higher doses of these nutrients are not necessary.

• **Zinc.** People suffering from rheumatoid arthritis often have low levels of the antioxidant zinc. In addition to eating more zinc-rich foods, consider a supplement of up to 30 to 45 milligrams a day. Some vitamin-mineral supplements contain this level of zinc.

• **Vitamin C.** The antioxidant vitamin C helps reduce inflammation associated with rheumatoid arthritis. (For more information on vitamin C, see "Supplements and Osteoarthritis," page 43.)

• **Fish oils.** Omega-3 polyunsaturated fatty acids have been shown to relieve inflammation and the symptoms of rheumatoid arthritis. A Danish study of fifty-one people with rheumatoid arthritis experienced significant improvement in stiffness and pain after twelve weeks on a daily dose of 3.6 grams of omega-3 polyunsaturated fatty acids. (The amount used in the study is equal to about one 8-ounce serving of salmon, mackerel, or herring.) It can take three to four months for the benefits to show up from a diet that regularly contains fish. The most widely available fish oil is EPA (eicosapentaenoic acid), which is available in health food stores. Another type is DHA (docosahexaenoic acid).

Supplements and Gout

Since diet and drug therapy are successful in treating most cases of gout, vitamin and mineral supplements aren't usually necessary. If you experience chronic gout, you might consider the following nutrition tips:

• **Vitamin C.** Megadoses of vitamin C can actually increase levels of uric acid in the blood. Skip the vitamin C supplements if you have gout.

• **Folic acid.** High levels of folic acid—roughly 10 milligrams per day—inhibit the enzyme responsible for producing uric acid. Caution: High levels of folic acid can interfere with the action of drugs used to treat epilepsy, in addition to masking the signs of vitamin B_{12} deficiency. Only take high doses of folic acid with your doctor's approval.

ARE YOU GETTING ENOUGH VITAMINS?

Eating a diet of vitamin-rich foods or taking vitamin and mineral supplements does not always guarantee that your body is absorbing and using all the nutrients made available to it. As people grow older, their bodies become less efficient at absorbing vitamins, especially folic acid and other B vitamins. In fact two people could consume the same foods and supplements and one could be fully nourished and the other nutrient deprived.

If what goes into your system isn't always what stays in your system, how can you be sure you're getting enough—but not too much—of the necessary nutrients? One possibility is to have a lab test done that measures the actual levels of vitamins and minerals in a small sample of blood.

Such tests usually cost about $300 and up. They can be done by a number of laboratories, but labs specializing in nutrition testing include Liberty Testing Laboratory in Brooklyn, New York; MetaMetrix in Atlanta; Pantox Laboratories in San Diego; and SpectraCell in Houston. Your doctor may prescribe a lab test for a particular nutrient, but most will not offer a full-spectrum nutrient profile.

Since there is considerable latitude in defining optimum nutrient levels, discuss the test results with your physician or a nutritionist, who can help you decide if any additional dietary adjustments might be necessary.

CHAPTER FIVE

Exercise: Work Out the Pain

If you hate exercise and you have arthritis, you may feel you have a perfect excuse for avoiding a workout. Alas, nothing could be farther from the truth. Exercise is a critical part of any arthritis treatment program. Without regular exercise arthritis pain will grow worse as joints stiffen and muscles weaken.

And don't forget the other multitudinous benefits of regular exercise: It improves circulation; lowers blood pressure; strengthens the heart and lungs; clears the arteries; releases endorphins, helping to lift depression; fights insomnia; and aids digestion. Add to the list a number of special benefits exercise offers the joints:

- Activities that put your joints through their full range of motion help keep them fully mobile.
- Exercise builds joint support by strengthening the muscles surrounding the joints.
- Regular movement increases the transportation of nutrients to the cartilage inside the joints.
- Weight-bearing exercise reduces your risk of developing

arthritis-related osteoporosis by helping to keep your bones dense and strong.
* Regular exercise helps control weight gain, which can make arthritis worse by adding to the load a joint must bear.

Of course vigorous exercise isn't possible for everyone with arthritis, but some type of exercise can be helpful for virtually everyone. A physical therapist can help you design an exercise program that suits your needs, lifestyle, and abilities.

Use It or Lose It

In the past, people with arthritis were encouraged to rest and restrict their activity. Not surprisingly long periods of inactivity lead to loss of flexibility and muscle weakness. What most arthritis sufferers need is a balance between regular exercise and appropriate rest.

A recent study conducted in the Netherlands shows that most exercise programs for people with arthritis are too conservative. People with rheumatoid arthritis are typically prescribed an exercise program consisting of isometric exercises (which place little pressure on the joints) and range-of-motion exercises (which keep the joints flexible). The researchers studied one hundred arthritic people, half of whom did the conventional combination of isometrics and range-of-motion exercises and the other half did intensive, dynamic exercise, such as bicycle riding, knee bending, walking at a fast pace, and step exercise. In the end those who performed the more vigorous, intense exercise routine had stronger muscles and greater joint mobility, in addition to being in better overall physical condition, than those who participated in the less challenging program.

Of course exercise can be overdone. Overzealous exercisers sometimes push themselves too hard and aggravate their condition. Use common sense: If it hurts, stop. Cut back on exercise and daily activities during flare-ups, when your joints are particularly painful and inflamed. Toughing it out and working through the pain is not only uncomfortable, it can also exacerbate joint deterioration by subjecting a damaged joint to undue stress.

The Importance of Rest

While exercise and regular activity are critical to the overall health of your joints, so is rest. As anyone with arthritis knows, some days are better than others. One of the most difficult tasks of learning to manage your arthritis is figuring out how to strike a balance between doing too much and doing too little. Ultimately you are the only one who knows how your joints feel and what you feel capable of doing on any given day.

One warning sign that you could be overworking yourself: You feel tired and your joints hurt for more than two hours after an activity. If possible, stop and rest before you tire; you'll be less likely to cause any damage from overuse. Also try ordering your routine so that you take on the most difficult tasks of the day when you tend to have the most energy.

Though it can be difficult to do, get plenty of sleep, try to incorporate several rest periods into your daily routine, and if possible, try to take a short nap during the day. Instead of mowing the lawn all at once, you may want to take a break and do it in two or three sessions. Try to be flexible: Listen to your body and allow yourself to change direction if you don't feel up to an activity you've planned.

If you need to rest a particular joint rather than to rest your entire body, you might consider using a splint to support and immobilize the joint. Splints are typically used on the hands and wrists of people with rheumatoid arthritis. They protect weak muscles, ligaments, and swollen joints. Because they keep the joint out of action, they often bring prompt relief while allowing the person to be otherwise active.

Most splints attach with Velcro straps. Three common types are resting splints (which prevent all movement of the affected joints), dynamic or working splints (which support the joint but allow some movement), and ulnar drift splints (which support the joints in the hands to prevent the fingers from drifting toward the little finger, as they often do as rheumatoid arthritis progresses).

If you believe your arthritis pain would be relieved through the use of a splint, contact a physical therapist, who can help fit you with the appropriate device.

Before You Get Started

Don't go it alone. Before jumping into an exercise program, talk it over with your physician. Some doctors want to do a complete medical evaluation and stress test, whereas others will just provide appropriate boundaries for a new program. In other cases your doctor may suggest that you work with a physical therapist to design the right exercise program for you. For information on finding a physical therapist, contact the American Physical Therapy Association, 1111 North Fairfax Street, Alexandria, Virginia 22314; (703) 684-2782.

Physical therapists practice in both hospitals and out-patient settings. You don't need your doctor's approval to work with a physical therapist, but your physical therapist may want to discuss your arthritic condition with your doctor before creating an exercise program for you.

A physical therapist will first assess your muscle strength and the range of motion of your joints. The exam may include an examination of your feet and a review of your walking gait for signs of any limp or imbalance. The therapist will then work with you to come up with a suitable exercise program. If you have mild arthritis, you may choose to work out on your own and visit the therapist only when your condition changes. However, if you have severe arthritis, you may want to exercise with the therapist several times a week.

Whether you consult a physical therapist or design an exercise program on your own, you'll have to come up with a schedule for getting regular workouts. It's more productive to exercise once or twice a day every day for fifteen or twenty minutes than to plan a longer, more ambitious workout that you never have time or energy to do.

Some people choose to work out first thing in the morning in order to overcome early-morning stiffness; others prefer to wait until the end of the day. When you work out is a matter of personal preference—as long as you do so regularly.

What Kind of Exercise?

You already exercise every day, even when you try not to. It takes exertion just to walk, bend, reach, lift, and carry yourself through the day. However, to build muscle strength, keep your joints flexible, and improve your overall physical condition, you almost certainly need a more challenging exercise routine than your daily activities.

In general, your daily exercise can be divided into two categories: *therapeutic* (exercises prescribed by your doctor or physical therapist based on your specific medical needs) and *recreational* (exercises and activities you choose to do for entertainment and to improve your overall health).

Your exercise routine should include a combination of exercises that achieve different goals. Ideally your workout should include the following types of exercise:

Range-of-Motion Exercises
These involve stretching a joint as far as it can go comfortably, then gently pushing just a bit farther. Done every day, these exercises maintain and build joint flexibility, in addition to relieving pain and increasing joint function. Flexing your fingers, bending your elbows, rotating your shoulders,

and raising and lowering your hands from the wrist are all examples of range-of-motion exercises.

Strengthening Exercises

These involve building the muscles to further stabilize and support weak joints. Muscles can be strengthened by performing isometric exercises (the muscle is tightened without moving the joint) or isotonic resistance exercises (light weights or other resistance is used as you move a muscle through its range of motion). Strengthening exercises are essential to rebuild muscles that have grown weak from disuse.

Endurance Exercises

Walking, swimming, biking, jogging, dancing, and aerobics are all examples of endurance exercise. These dynamic activities build endurance and improve aerobic condition, which improves the heart and circulatory system. (Swimming, especially in warm water, is an excellent option for people with arthritis because the water helps support the body's weight, minimizing stress on the joints.) Don't feel you have to baby your joints just because you have arthritis; appropriate activities can help heal the joints. For best results the activity should be continued for twenty to thirty minutes at least three times a week.

Exercise Tips

- **Get comfortable.** Wear loose and comfortable clothes that won't bind during exercise.
- **Begin slowly and build up exercise intensity slowly.** Too much, too fast can lead to pain and possible joint damage. A certain amount of discomfort may be inevitable if your arthritis is advanced, but pain that persists two hours or more after your workout is a sign that you've done too much.

- **Never hold your breath during exercise.** Keep your breathing slow and evenly paced.
- **Just do it.** For best results exercise every day. Sporadic exercise won't provide all the benefits. If you miss several days of exercise in a row, you may have to exercise at a lower intensity.
- **But don't overdo it.** Take it easy when it hurts. If your joints feel inflamed and painful, don't force them through the full range of motion. Don't give up on exercise, but don't force it. If your routine calls for three sets of five to ten repetitions, perhaps you should do only one set of exercises on a bad day. Listen to your body.
- **Keep your doctor informed.** If a joint becomes painful or you notice a limit in your range of motion, discuss the change with your doctor or physical therapist.
- **Keep your routine interesting.** If you're feeling bored, add background music or give yourself a reward for meeting your exercise goals.
- **Work out when you feel your best.** Whether it's first thing in the morning or after your first round of morning medication has kicked in, exercise when it feels right.
- **Avoid the heat.** If your joints feel hot, don't use them. Exercise can make a tender, swollen joint feel worse. Instead exercise any joints that don't feel irritated, then discuss the matter with your doctor or physical therapist.
- **Set realistic goals.** Don't plan on going out and walking a mile on your first day of exercise. Instead plan on walking—or performing the aerobic activity of your choice—for a fixed amount of time, say ten minutes. Then build the intensity gradually by increasing the amount of time you exercise.
- **Keep it smooth and steady.** Try to keep your breathing in pace with the repetitions of your exercise. Don't bounce or use jerky motions, which can add stress to the joints.

- **Log your progress.** Keep a daily record of your exercise routine and improvements.
- **Exercise with a friend.** An exercise partner or group can motivate you to get up and get moving, even when you don't feel the urge.
- **Schedule your exercise.** Make exercise a part of your daily routine. Don't allow other activities to interfere with your routine.
- **Massage yourself after exercise.** After a workout (or any time) you can use golf balls and tennis balls to exercise and massage achy muscles. By placing the ball in the palm of your hand and rubbing it against the affected area, you can give yourself a deep massage without straining your hands. Squeezing a tennis ball or rubber ball also strengthens the hands, fingers, and joints.

Exercise Throughout the Day

The benefits of exercise aren't limited to the activities performed during your prescribed workout. Every time you climb a flight of stairs, carry a bag of groceries, or lift the laundry out of the washer, you are getting exercise. The following tips may help you during your dawn-to-dusk daily workout:

1. **Sit up straight.** Good posture while sitting, standing, and walking can minimize pain and strengthen your muscles.

   - When sitting, keep your knees higher than your hips by resting your feet on a footstool or other object. Sit in straight-back chairs rather than rounding your back and sinking into a cushy couch.
   - When standing and walking, keep your spine lengthened, shoulders back, hips under. Pretend a string is

connected to the top of your head and is holding you
erect, like a marionette.

- When forced to stand for a prolonged period, shift
your weight and alternately raise one leg at a time and
rest it on a footstool to give your lower back a break.
(Keep this in mind when working in the kitchen.)

2. **Lift with care.** If you're forced to lift a heavy object,
squat down and lift with your knees rather than bending
over and lifting with your back. Don't try to lift a heavy
object above your waist.

3. **Get a good night's sleep.** Snooze on a firm mattress,
resting on your side, not on your stomach or back.

4. **Use a cane or walker if needed.** Don't be stubborn and
refuse to use a cane, walker, or wheelchair if your doctor or physical therapist recommends one. These devices help take the stress off your weight-bearing joints;
they can ease the pain, increase mobility, and prevent
some accidents.

- Learn to use a cane properly. A physical therapist
can help refine your skills, but a cane should be
used on the side opposite the affected joint. For
example, if your right hip, knee, or ankle is inflamed, hold the cane on your left side.

A Sample Routine for Building Strength and Mobility

When you start any exercise program, you should give
yourself plenty of time to get adjusted to the movement and
to get into condition to perform a full set of exercises. The
following suggested exercises can give you an idea of the
kind of stretches and strengthening exercises a physical therapist might prescribe, but there is no such thing as a one-

size-fits-all exercise routine for arthritis. To customize a workout to your specific needs, talk to your doctor or physical therapist.

These exercises should be done twice a day (morning and evening). At first expect to do only one or two repetitions of each exercise, then gradually increase the number of repetitions to a maximum of twenty per exercise session. Remember, the key to avoiding the pain of overuse is to increase your workload gradually.

If you experience pain while exercising, stop. Try the exercise again during the next session. If it still hurts, drop the exercise and consult a physical therapist.

The following routine includes exercises to improve both range of motion and strength. For a workout designed to build strength by lifting weights or using another form of resistance, consult a physical therapist.

Neck

1. *Look down:* Sit or stand, whichever is more comfortable. Keep your head straight and looking forward. Look directly down, bending at the neck. Try to rest your chin on your chest. Bend only as far as comfortable. Hold as you count to 10, then release.

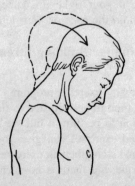

2. *Side to side:* Tilt your left ear toward your left shoulder without raising your shoulders. Hold as you count to 10, then shift and tilt your right ear toward your right shoulder and hold again.

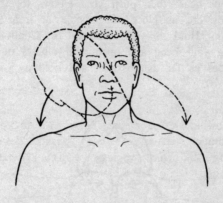

3. *Neck twist:* Smoothly turn your head to look over your left shoulder. Turn as far as possible without forcing. Hold as you count to 10, then gently turn your head in the opposite direction and hold again.

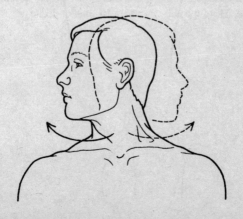

Shoulders

1. *Elbow touch:* Sit, stand, or lie down, whichever is most comfortable. Clasp your hands behind your head, then push your elbows together until they arc as close as possible in front of your chin. Hold as you count to 10. Continue holding your head and open your elbows out to the sides as far as possible, and hold as you count to 10.

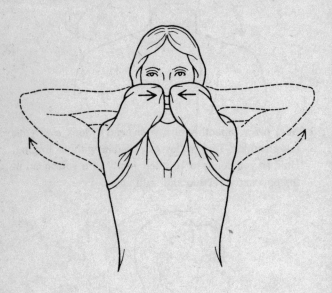

2. *Spread your wings:* Stand with your arms at your sides. Gently reach your arms behind your back as far as you can. Hold and count to 10.

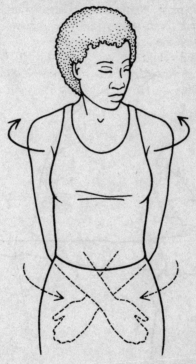

3. *Hands up:* Stand with your arms straight out in front of you. Raise both arms straight overhead, reaching for the sky. Hold as you count to 10.

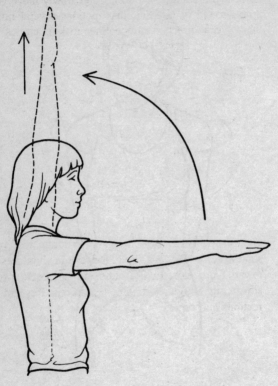

4. *Fly away:* Stand with your arms at your sides. Raise both arms directly out from your sides and lift them over your head. Keep your arms as straight as possible and hold as you count to 10. Relax and slowly move your arms around in large circular motions several times, then reverse direction and continue making circles.

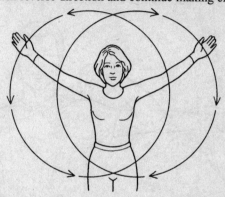

5. *Shoulder rolls:* Either sitting or standing, roll your shoulders in a forward circle. Raise your shoulders up toward your ears, then around to your back. Move slowly and smoothly for five repetitions. Reverse directions and repeat.

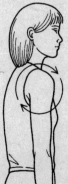
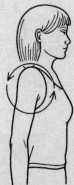

Elbows and Arms

1. *Shoulder touch:* Stand with your arms at your sides. Bend your arms at the elbows, touching your shoulders, then straighten your arm, holding it directly out to your side. Repeat five times.

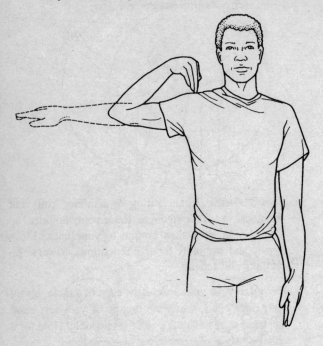

2. *Forearm roll:* Stand with your elbows at your waist and your forearms extended. Turn your arms so that your palms are facing up, then rotate so that your palms are turned downward. Rotate your palms as far as possible in each direction, holding for a count of 10 in each direction before reversing.

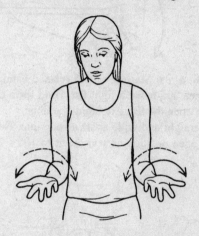

Wrists, Hands, and Fingers

1. *Wrist flex:* Rest your arm on the edge of a table. Using your right hand, touch the fingers of your left hand and bend your wrist back as far as possible. Hold for a count of 10. Repeat with the opposite hand.

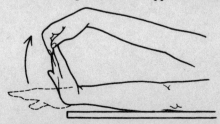

2. *Wrist bend:* Rest your arm on a table with your wrist just over the edge. Use your right hand to bend your hand as far down as possible. Hold for a count of 10, then repeat with the opposite hand.

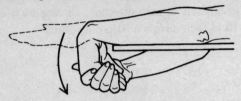

3. *Make a fist:* Starting with a relaxed hand, close your fingers and make a tight fist. Hold for a count of 10, then open the fist, extending the fingers to make them as straight and wide apart as possible. Hold again in the open position as you count to 10.

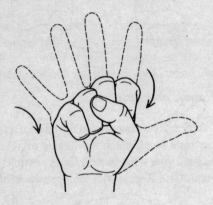

4. *Get a grip:* Using a foam or sponge ball (not a hard rubber ball) slightly larger than a tennis ball, squeeze as tightly as possible. Hold for a count of 10, then release and straighten your fingers.

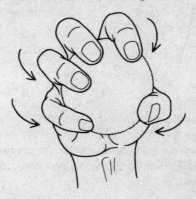

5. *Bowing fingers:* One finger at a time, curl each finger down toward your palm, one joint at a time. If necessary, use the opposite hand to help move the appropriate finger. Repeat with the opposite hand.

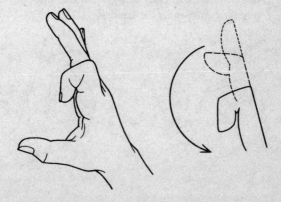

6. *Flat on the table:* Place your palms flat on a table and press firmly. Hold the position as you count to 10. Alternate hands and repeat.

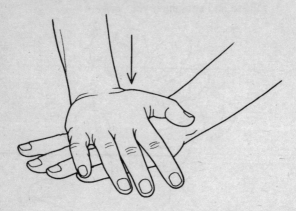

7. *Everything's A-OK:* Touch your thumb and pointer finger together to form the letter *O*. Repeat the motion, using the thumb and each finger in the hands, taking care to form a well-rounded letter with each finger. This exercise helps with the grasping and pinching motion in the hands.

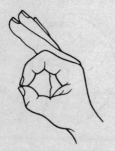 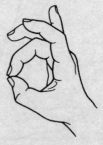

8. *Spread 'em:* Hold your hands up and spread your fingers as far apart as possible. Hold as you count to 10. Then close them together as tightly as possible. Again, hold as you count to 10.

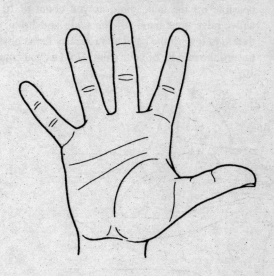

9. *Thumbs up:* Place your hands flat on your lap or on a table. Push your thumbs away from your hands as far as possible; hold as you count to 10. Bring your thumb in to your hand, then try to lift it as far as possible off the table; hold as you count to 10. Finally, raise your hand off the table and bring your thumb in toward the hand and reach as far as possible toward the middle of your palm. Hold as you count to 10.

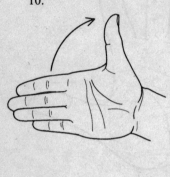

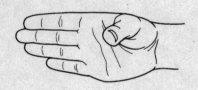

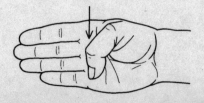

Hips

1. *Knees up:* Lying in bed or on the floor, bend your right knee up to your chest. Grasp your leg behind the knee and pull your leg in to your body. Hold as you count to 10, then repeat with the opposite leg. Then pull both knees up to your chest together and again hold as you count to 10. Gently rock from side to side while rolled up in a ball.

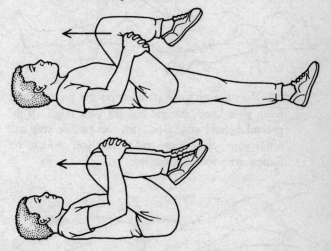

2. *Hip roll:* Lie on your back on the bed or floor. Keep one leg flat and bend the other so that your knee is pointed up to the ceiling. Rotate the leg out to one side, then hold as you count to 10. Move your leg in the opposite direction and hold again. Repeat with the opposite leg.

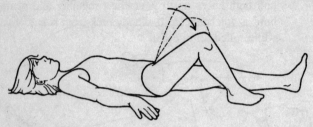

3. *Hip flex:* Lie on your stomach on the floor or bed. Keep your knees straight and lift your thigh off the ground behind you. Don't lift too far, or you will rotate your pelvis. Raise and hold as you count to 10. Repeat with the opposite leg.

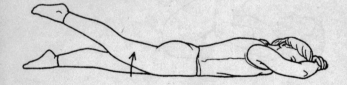

4. *Butterfly feet:* Lie on your back on the floor or bed. Turn your knees and feet inward, trying to touch your toes together while keeping your legs flat. Hold as you count to 10. Rotate your knees and feet outward, trying to touch your toes to the ground. Hold as you count to 10.

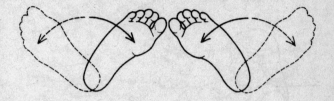

Knees and Legs

1. *Get a leg up:* Sit in a chair with your feet flat on the floor. Raise one leg and rest it on a table or another chair that is of comfortable height. Keep your leg as straight as possible, flex your toes back, and hold as you count to 10.

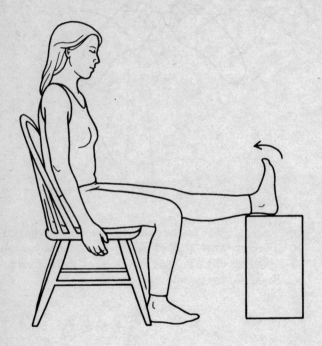

2. *Leg raise:* Lie on your back on the floor or bed. Bend one knee, leaving the foot flat on the ground. Raise the opposite leg straight up as far as you can, while keeping your back pressed firmly against the ground. Do not allow your back to arch. When your leg has been raised as far as possible, hold for a count of 10, then repeat with the opposite leg.

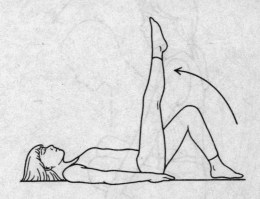

3. *Knee flex:* Lie on your stomach on the floor or bed. Bend one knee, reaching your ankle as far as you can toward your back. Hold as you count to 10, then release and repeat with the opposite leg.

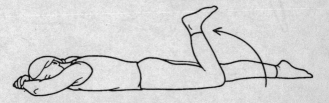

4. *Stretch it out:* Sit on the floor with your legs crossed in front of you. Reach down and hold your feet with your hands. Lean forward slowly, gradually stretching the muscles in your back, legs, and hips. Hold as you count to 10.

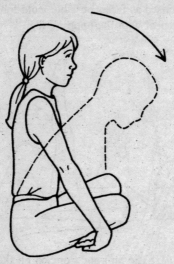

Ankles and Feet

1. *Toe lifts:* Sit up straight in a chair with your bare feet flat on the floor. Raise your toes as high as possible while keeping your heels on the floor. Hold as you count to 10. Relax, then keep your toes on the floor and lift your heels as high as possible, and again hold as you count to 10.

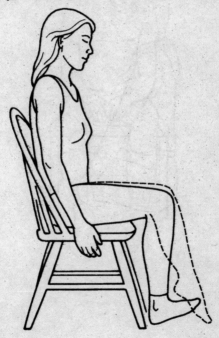

2. *Foot curls:* Sitting in a chair, curl your toes and roll the weight of your foot to the outside, turning the soles of your feet so that they face each other.

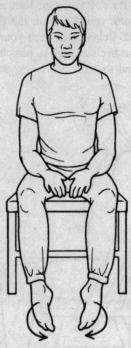

3. *Ankle rolls:* Sitting in a chair, lift one foot at a time and rotate your ankle in a complete circle. Reverse directions and rotate again.

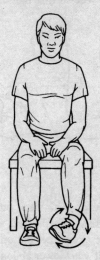

4. *Over the edge:* Stand on the edge of a stair or step. Bend your toes over the edge and press down firmly. Hold as you count to 10, then relax.

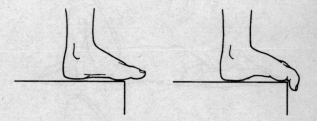

5. *Throw down the towel:* Sit in a chair with your bare feet resting on a towel on the floor. Curl your toes and use them to gather the towel under your feet.

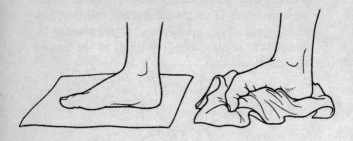

Back

1. *Pelvic tilt:* Lie on your back on the floor or in bed. Relax and raise your arms over your head. Bend your knees and keep your feet flat on the ground. Tighten the muscles of your lower abdomen and buttocks and flatten your back against the floor or bed. Press flat on the floor as you hold for a count of 10.

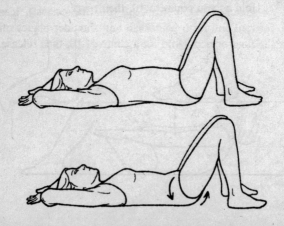

2. *Building bridges:* Lie on your back on the floor or in bed. Bend your knees and keep your feet and palms flat on the floor. Slowly raise your buttocks off the ground 4 to 6 inches. Do not arch your back; instead press the small of your back flat and roll your buttocks up and off the ground. Hold as you count to 10, then slowly release, easing yourself to the ground vertebra by vertebra.

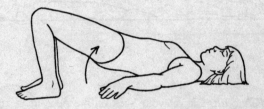

3. *Modified sit-up:* Lie on your back on the floor or in bed. Bend your knees and keep your feet flat on the floor. With your arms locked behind your neck (the hardest), crossed in front of your chest (a bit easier), or stretched out in front of you (the easiest), lean forward and raise your head and shoulder blades off the floor or bed. Hold for a count of 10, then release.

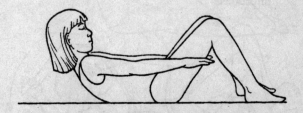

4. *Back stretch:* Lie on your stomach on the floor or bed with your arms straight down at your sides. Raise your head, arms, and legs off the floor as far as possible, keeping your legs straight. (Don't worry if you can't raise yourself too far off the ground; this exercise will help build both flexibility and back strength.) Hold as you count to 10, then relax.

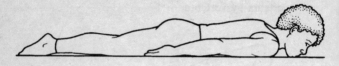

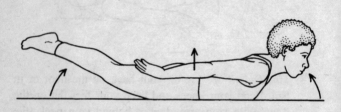

5. *Do the twist:* Lie on your back on the floor or bed. Bend your knees and keep your feet flat on the floor. Turn your arms and head to the right while shifting your knees and legs to the left, giving yourself a nice torso stretch. Hold as you count to 10, then reverse directions.

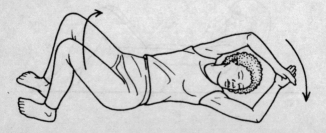

6. *Bicycling:* Lie on your back on the floor or bed. Fold your hands and slip them under your buttocks for support. Raise your legs in the air and make a motion like you are pedaling a bicycle through five to ten cycles.

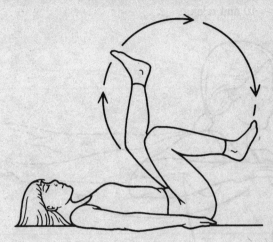

Chest

1. *Open up:* Stand tall. Bend your arms and raise your elbows at your sides to shoulder height. Straighten your arms and reach backward. Hold as you count to 10 and relax.

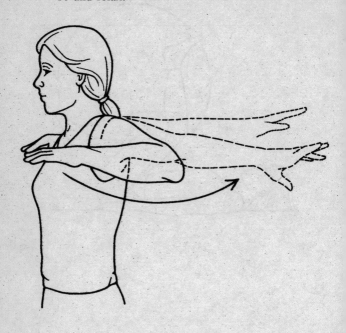

2. *Arm swing:* Stand in a relaxed position with your arms down and crossed in front of you. In a controlled motion, swing your arms up and over your head, reaching out as far as possible. Inhale as you raise your arms and exhale as you lower them.

CHAPTER SIX

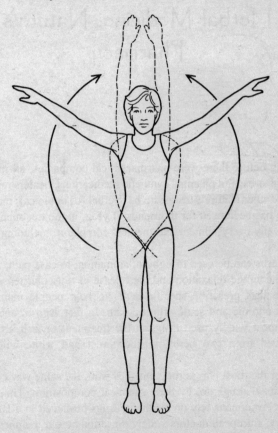

Herbal Medicine: Nature's Pharmacy

Long before there were pharmaceutical companies, all-night drugstores, and patented synthetic medications, healers relied on Mother Nature's drugs: herbs. Herbal (or botanical) medicine has been used for thousands of years in the treatment of virtually every ailment and medical complaint, including arthritis.

Herbs can be used to fight inflammation, to ease pain, and to encourage relaxation and the release of muscular tension. Herbalists prescribe specific herbs to help people manage both chronic and acute arthritic pain. In fact aspirin, one of the most widely used drugs in the treatment of arthritis, is derived from two herbs, meadowsweet and white willow bark.

For the most part herbal remedies work the same way conventional drugs do, by their chemical composition. Though most Americans rely on synthetic drugs produced in a laboratory, European doctors widely prescribe herbal treatments. For example when treating depression German doctors recommend Saint John's wort, an herb, for more than half of their patients.

In the treatment of arthritis, herbs offer one distinct advantage over traditional drugs: While aspirin and other pain-relievers and antiinflammatory drugs can take the edge off the pain and reduce swelling, they won't help stop the progression of the disease, and in some cases can make matters worse. Herbal treatments, on the other hand, don't merely mask the symptoms of arthritis; they actually help the body heal itself.

Because of their sometimes potent healing effects, herbal medicines, like all medicines, deserve our respect. Just because herbs are natural does not mean that they are benign. When used incorrectly or at excessively high doses, herbs, like any drugs, can have negative—and sometimes dangerous—side effects. Before taking any herbs at medicinal strengths, discuss the issue with your medical practitioner.

The herbal remedies described here can have side effects in some people; any common negative side effects are listed with each entry. At the dosages listed the herbal treatments are safe, but to minimize the risk of unpleasant side effects, start with the lowest possible dose and then gradually increase either the strength of the type of preparation used or its frequency of use, up to the limits stated here. In all cases, if you're using a commercial product, follow the dosage directions on the package label.

Herbal remedies have traditionally been available in health food stores, but increasingly they are showing up in supermarkets and pharmacies. Browse your local stores, check the Yellow Pages for listings of health food stores in your area, or refer to the "Resources" section at the end of this chapter for information on mail-order companies that sell herbs.

The herbs listed in this chapter are single herbs rather than formulas, or blends of herbs designed to act synergistically to achieve specific results for specific individuals. Herbal formulas may be available commercially, otherwise they can be prepared by a professional.

Using Herbs

Herbal medicines can be made from a number of different parts of the plant, including the flowers, roots, leaves, seeds, bark, and rhizomes. Thousands of years of trial and error by herbalists and healers have refined the appropriate "recipes" for herbal medicines. Though only a small fraction of the world's plants have been tested for their medicinal potential, there are approximately one thousand herbs available in the United States to treat everything from arthritis to heart disease.

Herbal medicines come in a variety of forms, including:

- **Teas:** Made by steeping about 1 teaspoon of dried herbs in 1 cup of boiling water for 5 minutes or so, then straining. Most herbal teas are not strong enough to provide medicinal value.
- **Infusions:** Made like tea, but the herbs are steeped for 20 to 30 minutes, so the resulting liquid is more potent.
- **Decoctions:** Made like infusions, only the bark or roots of the herbs are simmered with the lid on (never boiled), rather than merely steeped, for 20 to 30 minutes (or sometimes longer) to prevent the loss of valuable components as well as to keep the liquid from evaporating.
- **Tinctures:** Made by soaking herbs in an alcohol solution for a specified period of time (from several hours to several days).
- **Extracts:** Made by distilling the alcohol from a tincture, leaving a more potent concentrate behind.
- **Powders:** Made by removing all moisture from an extract, then grinding the solid herbal concentrate into granules or powders, which can then be shaped into capsules or tablets.

Most of the herbal treatments described here involve infusions or decoctions, which may have a sharp, bitter taste. You can try to mask the unpleasant flavor with sugar, honey, lemon, fruit juice, or even flavored tea mix. If you don't want to prepare your own herbs, tinctures and extracts are commercially available at health food stores and some drugstores.

WARNING: Do not use herbs if you are pregnant or nursing. Babies lack some of the liver enzymes needed to detoxify chemicals in herbs. Contact a qualified herbalist or naturopathic physician for more information.

Useful Herbs for Arthritis

Alfalfa (Medicago sativa)
ALSO KNOWN AS: Buffalo grass, Chilean clover.
USES: Alfalfa is often used to alleviate inflammation and pain associated with arthritis and rheumatic disease. It may also help reduce cholesterol levels.
PREPARATION: For an infusion, add 1 to 2 teaspoons dried herb to 1 cup boiling water. Steep for 15 minutes. Let cool and drink up to 3 cups a day. Tinctures and extracts are commercially available; follow package directions.
SIGNS OF OVERDOSE: Stomach upset, diarrhea.
WARNING: Use only alfalfa leaves for medicinal purposes. Alfalfa sprouts can spruce up a salad or sandwich but they have no medicinal benefits. Alfalfa seeds, on the other hand, contain a toxic amino acid that can cause a blood disorder if consumed in large quantities.

Angelica (Anglica atropurpurea)
ALSO KNOWN AS: Wild celery, masterwort.
USES: Angelica has antiinflammatory effects that have made it a favorite arthritis treatment in Asian cultures for centuries. It also helps relieve digestive complaints.
PREPARATION: For a decoction, use 1 teaspoon powdered root

per cup of water. Bring to a boil, simmer 2 minutes, then remove from heat and let stand for 15 minutes. Drink up to 2 cups a day. Tinctures and extracts are commercially available; follow package directions.

POSSIBLE UNINTENDED EFFECT: Skin rash when exposed to sunlight.

WARNING: Angelica can stimulate uterine contractions; it should not be used by pregnant women.

Barberry *(Berberis vulgaris)*

ALSO KNOWN AS: Berberry, jaundice berry.

USES: This powerful herb fights bacterial infection, boosts the immune system, and may also reduce inflammation. Research has shown that barberry is stronger than some pharmaceutical antibiotics.

PREPARATION: For a decoction, simmer ½ teaspoon powdered root bark in 1 cup water for 20 to 30 minutes. Allow to cool and drink up to 1 cup a day. Tinctures and extracts are commercially available; follow package directions.

SIGNS OF OVERDOSE: Nausea, vomiting, drop in blood pressure.

WARNING: This herb should not be used by pregnant women, since it can stimulate uterine contractions.

Black Cohosh *(Cimicifuga racemosa)*

ALSO KNOWN AS: Snakeroot, squawroot.

USES: For centuries the Algonquian Indians used decoctions of black cohosh to treat arthritis, as well as menstrual and menopausal discomfort.

PREPARATION: For a decoction, simmer ½ teaspoon powdered root or 1 teaspoon cut and sifted root per cup of water for 30 minutes. Let cool and drink 2 tablespoons every few hours for up to 1 cup a day. Tinctures and extracts are commercially available; follow package directions.

SIGNS OF OVERDOSE: Dizziness, nausea, abdominal pain, headache.

WARNING: This is a potent herb; it should be used only under the supervision of a medical professional.

Black Haw *(Viburnum prunifolium)*

ALSO KNOWN AS: Viburnum.

USES: The bark of this herb has been used to ease arthritis pain, as well as prevent miscarriage and menstrual cramps.

PREPARATION: For a decoction, use 2 teaspoons dried bark per cup of water. Simmer 20 to 30 minutes, then let cool. Drink up to 2 cups a day. Tinctures and extracts are commercially available; follow package directions.

SIGNS OF OVERDOSE: Upset stomach, nausea, vomiting, ringing in the ears.

WARNING: Black haw can cause birth defects; pregnant women should not use this herb.

Boneset *(Eupatorium perfoliatum)*

ALSO KNOWN AS: Feverwort.

USES: This herb does not mend fractured bones, but it can help fight inflammation, making it a useful herb in the treatment of some forms of arthritis. The herb can induce sweating and is widely used to treat fever and fever-producing illnesses.

PREPARATION: For an infusion, use 1 to 2 teaspoons dried leaves per cup of boiling water. Steep for 20 to 30 minutes. Let cool and drink up to 3 cups a day. Tinctures and extracts are commercially available; follow package directions.

SIGNS OF OVERDOSE: Nausea, vomiting, diarrhea.

WARNING: People with a history of alcoholism or liver disease should not use this herb.

Boswellia *(Boswellia serrata)*

ALSO KNOWN AS: Boswellic acid.

USES: The gum resin from this large, branching tree from India is used in the treatment of arthritis because of its anti-

inflammatory effects and because it improves the blood supply to the joints.

PREPARATION: Available at health food stores as capsules; 400
milligrams, three times daily, is the common dosage. Tinctures and extracts are commercially available; follow package
directions.

UNINTENDED EFFECTS: None known.

Burdock *(Arctium lappa)*

ALSO KNOWN AS: Great burdock.

USES: This herb used to be called a blood cleanser because it
stimulates the lymphatic system to release toxins. It does not
act directly on the inflammation or discomfort of arthritis,
but can be added to an arthritis formula. A compress of hot
burdock can be used to soothe the swelling of arthritis.

PREPARATION: For a compress, prepare tea using 1 teaspoon
herb with 1 cup water. Soak a clean towel in the tea and
apply directly to the affected joint. Tinctures and extracts are
commercially available; follow package directions.

UNINTENDED EFFECTS: None when the herb is used as a compress.

Chamomile *(Anthemis nobilis)*

ALSO KNOWN AS: Ground apple, anthemis.

USES: This herb promotes relaxation, which can help arthritis
sufferers who need to unwind and relieve stress.

PREPARATION: Use 2 to 3 heaping teaspoons of herb per cup of
boiling water. Steep for 15 minutes. Drink up to 3 cups a
day. Tinctures and extracts are commercially available; follow package directions.

SIGNS OF OVERDOSE: Nausea and vomiting. It can cause allergic
reactions in people who are allergic to pollens.

Coriander (or Cilantro) (Coriandrum sativum)

ALSO KNOWN AS: Chinese parsley.

USES: Because of its antiinflammatory properties, coriander has been used to treat arthritis (though it is best known as a digestive aid). The herb is often used in herbal formulas, prepared by a professional herbalist.

SIGNS OF OVERDOSE: Stomach upset.

Devil's Claw (Harpagophytum porcumbens)

ALSO KNOWN AS: No alternative names.

USES: Devil's claw has both antiinflammatory and analgesic effects; it contains a chemical, harpagoside, that reduces joint inflammation. It has also been shown to lower uric acid levels, making it useful in the treatment of gout.

PREPARATION: For an infusion, add 1 to 2 teaspoons dried herb to 1 cup boiling water. Steep for 15 minutes. Let cool and drink up to 2 cups a day. Tinctures and extracts are commercially available; follow package directions.

SIGNS OF OVERDOSE: Stomach upset.

WARNING: This herb should not be used by pregnant women.

Echinacea (Echinacea augustifolia)

ALSO KNOWN AS: Purple coneflower.

USES: The Plains Indians used echinacea tea to treat arthritis, as well as to boost the immune system and fight infection. Many forms of arthritis cause the breakdown of hyaluronic acid, which lubricates the joints. Echinacea protects this chemical and fights inflammation.

PREPARATION: To make a decoction, simmer 2 teaspoons of root per cup of water for 30 to 60 minutes. Drink up to 3 cups a day. Tinctures and extracts are commercially available; follow package directions.

SIGNS OF OVERDOSE: Tingling on the tongue, stomach upset, and diarrhea.

WARNING: This herb should not be used by people with severe arthritis, unless recommended by a qualified herbalist.

Eucalyptus *(Eucalyptus globulus)*

ALSO KNOWN AS: Gum tree, Australian fever tree.

USES: Best known for its use in the treatment of colds, flu, and bronchitis, eucalyptus ointment also helps relieve pain associated with arthritis and rheumatism.

PREPARATION: Look for a prepared ointment in health food stores, or prepare your own by adding several drops of eucalyptus oil to a teaspoon of olive oil, and apply it directly to the affected joints. Tinctures and extracts are commercially available; follow package directions.

UNINTENDED EFFECTS: Possible skin rash in people with sensitive skin.

Fenugreek *(Trigonella foenum-graecum)*

ALSO KNOWN AS: Greek hay, finigreek.

USES: This herb helps fight inflammation, making it useful in the treatment of arthritis. It also reduces cholesterol levels.

PREPARATION: For a decoction, simmer 2 teaspoons crushed seeds per cup of water for 20 to 30 minutes; be sure to cover the pot. Let cool and drink up to 3 cups a day. Tinctures and extracts are commercially available; follow package directions.

SIGNS OF OVERDOSE: Stomach upset.

WARNING: The herb can stimulate uterine contractions; pregnant women should not use it. Also women who have been told not to use contraceptive pills or who have a history of breast cancer should not use fenugreek.

Gentian *(Gentiana lutea)*

ALSO KNOWN AS: Bitterwort, bitter root.

USES: Chinese herbalists have long prescribed gentian in the treatment of arthritis. It also stimulates digestion, especially when taken before meals.

PREPARATION: For a decoction, boil 1 teaspoon powdered root in 3 cups water for 30 minutes. Let cool, then drink 1 tablespoon before meals. Tinctures and extracts are commercially available; follow package directions.

SIGNS OF OVERDOSE: Nausea and vomiting.

Ginger *(Zingiber officinale)*

ALSO KNOWN AS: African ginger.

USES: In addition to its use in controlling motion sickness and nausea, ginger helps relieve inflammation associated with arthritis.

PREPARATION: To make ginger tea, use 2 teaspoons powdered or grated root per cup of water. Simmer for 20 to 30 minutes. Drink up to 2 cups a day.

In addition, a compress made of hot ginger can ease the pain and tension of stiff joints. To make a compress, grate 4 ounces raw ginger and put it in a clean cotton sock. Bring 1/2 gallon of water to a boil, then remove from the heat and add the sock, filled with ginger. When the water turns yellow, after 5 to 10 minutes, soak a towel in the liquid and apply to the painful joints. Leave the ginger-soaked towel on the joint for 15 to 20 minutes, rewetting it as necessary to keep the towel warm. Another option: The decoction can be used as a compress as well. Tinctures and extracts are commercially available; follow package directions.

SIGNS OF OVERDOSE: Heartburn.

Horsetail *(Equisetum arvense)*

ALSO KNOWN AS: Bottle brush, corncob plant, pewterwort.

USES: This marsh-growing herb absorbs gold that is dissolved in water. Doctors often prescribe gold in the treatment of rheumatoid arthritis, and Chinese herbalists have long recommended horsetail for arthritis.

PREPARATION: For an infusion, use 1 to 2 teaspoons dried herb per cup of water. Steep 10 minutes. Let cool and drink up to 2 cups a day. Tinctures and extracts are commercially available; follow package directions.

SIGNS OF OVERDOSE: Fever, weight loss.

WARNING: Horsetail contains high levels of selenium, which can cause birth defects, so pregnant women should avoid this herb.

Juniper (Juniperus communis)

ALSO KNOWN AS: Geneva.

USES: This herb reduces inflammation and is widely prescribed in Europe for the treatment of arthritis. It is also used in the treatment of premenstrual syndrome and high blood pressure.

PREPARATION: For a decoction, use 1 teaspoon crushed berries per cup of water and simmer for 20 to 30 minutes. Let cool and drink up to 2 cups a day. Tinctures and extracts are commercially available; follow package directions.

SIGNS OF OVERDOSE: Diarrhea, kidney pain, blood or protein in the urine.

WARNING: Juniper can damage the kidneys in high doses; people with kidney infection or damage should not use this herb.

Licorice (Glycyrrhiza glabra)

ALSO KNOWN AS: No alternative names.

USES: For thousands of years licorice has been used in the treatment of arthritis, as well as other illnesses, because of its antiinflammatory properties.

PREPARATION: For a decoction, gently boil ½ teaspoon powdered licorice with 1 cup water for 10 minutes. Drink no more than 1 cup per day. Tinctures and extracts are commercially available; follow package directions.

SIGNS OF OVERDOSE: Water retention and changes in metabolism.

Meadowsweet *(Filipendula ulmaria)*

ALSO KNOWN AS: Bridewort, queen-of-the-meadow.

USES: Herbalists have long recommended meadowsweet to treat arthritis; the herb contains salicin, the powerful analgesic and antiinflammatory agent found in aspirin.

PREPARATION: For an infusion, use 1 to 2 teaspoons dried herb per cup of boiling water. Steep for 20 to 30 minutes. Let cool and drink up to 3 cups a day. Tinctures and extracts are commercially available; follow package directions.

SIGNS OF OVERDOSE: Stomach upset, ringing in the ears.

WARNING: Meadowsweet has been associated with birth defects; pregnant women should not use it.

Turmeric *(Curcuma longa)*

ALSO KNOWN AS: Curcuma.

USES: Curcumin, a healing chemical in the herb turmeric, helps kill bacteria, improve digestion, and it has antiinflammatory properties used to treat arthritis. In fact curcumin has been shown to be as effective as cortisone at fighting acute inflammation.

PREPARATION: For an infusion, add 1 teaspoon turmeric powder to 1 cup warm water. Drink up to 3 cups a day. Tinctures and extracts are commercially available; follow package directions.

SIGNS OF OVERDOSE: Stomach upset.

White Willow *(Salix alba)*

ALSO KNOWN AS: Salicin willow.

USES: Aspirin was first developed from a chemical derived from the bark of the white willow. This herb helps relieve pain and reduce inflammation.

PREPARATION: For an infusion, soak 1 teaspoon powdered bark per cup of cold water for 8 hours. Strain and drink up to 3 cups a day. If you don't want to wait that long, prepare a decoction by adding 1 teaspoon powdered bark per cup of water and simmering for 30 to 60 minutes. Tinctures and extracts are commercially available; follow package directions.

SIGNS OF OVERDOSE: Stomach upset, nausea, ringing in the ears.

WARNING: Children should not be given aspirin due to the risk of developing Reye's syndrome, a potentially fatal disease of the brain and kidneys. Do not give white willow bark to children under age sixteen.

RESOURCES: HERBAL MEDICINE

Herbal medicine is used by many naturopathic physicians and acupuncturists. However, there is no separate certification or licensing process specifically for herbalists.

For information on herbal medicine and referrals to practitioners in your area, contact:

The American Herbalists Guild
P.O. Box 1683
Soquel, California 95073
(408) 464-2441

Additional publications, newsletters, and books on herbal medicine are available from:

The American Botanical Council
P.O. Box 201660
Austin, Texas 78720
(512) 331-8868
(800) 373-7105

Herb Research Foundation
1007 Pearl Street, Suite 200
Boulder, Colorado 80302
(303) 449-2265

Sources of herbal mail-order supplies include:

Earth's Harvest
2557 N.W. Division
Gresham, Oregon 97030
(800) 428-3308

East Earth Trade Winds
P.O. Box 493151
Redding, California 96049-3151
(800) 258-6878
(916) 241-6878 in California

Eclectic Institute
14385 Lusted Road
Sandy, Oregon 97055
(800) 332-HERB

Herb-Pharm
P.O. Box 116
William, Oregon 97544
(503) 846-6262

Herbs of Grace
Division of School of Natural Medicine
P.O. Box 7369
Boulder, Colorado 80306-7369
(303) 443-4882

Meridian Traditional Herbal Products
44 Linden Street
Brookline, Massachusetts 02146
(800) 356-6003
(617) 739-2636 in Massachusetts

McZand Herbal, Inc.
P.O. Box 5312
Santa Monica, California 90409
(310) 822-0500

Nature's Way Products, Inc.
10 Mountain Springs Parkway
Springville, Utah 84663
(801) 489-1520

Windriver Herbs
P.O. Box 3876
Jackson, Wyoming 83001
(800) 903-HERB

CHAPTER SEVEN

Acupressure: Hands-on Healing

The human touch can heal. The ancient art of acupressure involves the use of touch to stimulate the body's natural ability to heal itself. In the practice of acupressure the tips of the fingers are used to press firmly on certain key points on the body. The pressure relaxes the surrounding muscles and stimulates the blood flow to the affected area. (Acupuncture uses the same network of key points as acupressure, except that ultra-fine needles pierce the skin at the trigger spots to stimulate the area.)

Acupressure, a technique that has been used by the Chinese for more than five thousand years, is safe, effective, easy, and nontoxic. Of course acupressure cannot "cure" rheumatic disease or restore worn-down bone and cartilage, but it can ease arthritis pain by relaxing the muscles and soft tissues to the point that the bones no longer grind against one another, causing pain. Acupressure is not intended to replace traditional medical care for most patients, but it can help many people with arthritis combat pain without dependence on pain-relievers and other drugs.

Understanding Acupressure

No one knows the actual origins of acupressure as a method of healing, but one popular myth holds that the Chinese accidentally discovered the technique during battle, when soldiers pierced by arrows experienced sudden relief from long-standing pain or illness in another part of the body. According to this story, after that initial observation, ancient Chinese healers began to look for relationships between pain relief and stimulation of certain key points on the body, and the practice of acupressure was born.

Of course we will never know whether the technique was inspired on the battlefield or by keen observation alone. What we do know, however, is that over thousands of years, healers have observed and carefully recorded the relationship between stimulating certain points and relieving pain in distant parts of the body. Over the centuries this time-honored technique has been refined through trial and error and careful observation. Today acupressure practitioners rely on detailed maps that include hundreds of pressure points throughout the body. Gone is the guesswork: Practitioners now know the healing effects of stimulating these points.

These acupressure points are locations on the body that are particularly sensitive to the bioelectrical impulses triggered by touch. The points lie along pathways throughout the body that carry "essential life energy" (called *qi* or *chi* in Chinese). When a person is healthy, this life energy flows smoothly throughout the body. When someone suffers from an illness or injury, such as arthritis, the energy is blocked or deficient. The disruption of the energy leads to an imbalance between the *yin* (passive energy) and *yang* (active energy).

In addition the acupressure points correlate with key spots where muscular tension tends to accumulate. Stress or tension can cause a cramp or knot in a muscle, which in turn can block the flow of life energy and cause the body to fall out of balance. Acupressure helps relax the muscles and stimulate blood flow, which can renew the flow of *qi* throughout the body. The additional blood flow also helps oxygenate the area, which can further promote healing.

Some of the profound relaxation accompanying acupressure may be due to the release of endorphins, the body's natural pain-relieving chemicals. When key points are stimulated, the body releases a shot of feel-good endorphins. Another popular theory is that the technique works by transmitting new pain impulses, which block the pathway for the pain signals resulting from the arthritis. This "pain gateway" theory suggests that the stimulation caused by the acupressure "closes the gates" of the body's pain-signaling system. The brain can process only so many signals at one time, and the acupressure stimulation may override the pain signals sent by the joints.

There are two types of acupressure points: local points (where the pain occurs) and trigger points (a point far from the site where the pain occurs). These trigger points lie along a network of electrical channels (called meridians) that run throughout the body. Acupressure healers have identified twelve major meridians, each named after or corresponding to a different organ, such as Large Intestine, Small Intestine, or Bladder. The meridians connect the acupressure points throughout the body, a sort of wiring system for the flow of the body's life energy or bioelectrical impulses. Stimulating one spot in the network can stimulate other points along the same pathway or meridian.

Practicing Acupressure

Acupressure isn't as complex or intimidating as it might seem if you're a beginner. Each of the body's 365 acupressure points has been named, numbered, and plotted on a map of physical landmarks, such as joints and indentations in the bones. Most of the points (or *tsubos*) lie beneath the major muscle groups, in the hollows of the bones, or along the bone structure. You'll know you've located the appropriate spot if you feel a tingle or electrical impulse when you apply direct pressure.

Once you've isolated the target point, use your thumbs, middle finger, palms, or the side of your hands to apply firm, steady pressure. Hold your finger at a right angle to the body. Begin with a light touch and gradually increase the pressure until you feel a deep, even pressure. Don't press so forcefully that you feel pain. You should build up the pressure slowly and steadily, without poking or jabbing.

Just one minute of steady pressure can promote healing and calm the nervous system, but three to five minutes of firm pressure usually works best. Whenever possible, work on both the right and left sides at the same time to maintain balance in your body. If your hand gets tired during an acupressure session, ease up on the pressure, shake out your hands to relax the muscles, then try again if you wish.

The more relaxed you feel, the more successful your acupressure session will be. Practice deep breathing to keep the body relaxed and fully oxygenated (see "Breathing," page 141). Focus on the healing process and imagine your painful joints relaxing and letting go of the pain. Once you become more familiar with the key acupressure points for arthritis, you will be able to lie down on your bed and close your eyes during your acupressure session, providing for even deeper relaxation.

While acupressure can provide immediate relief of some arthritic pain, long-term results require regular practice. Plan on spending twenty minutes or so working through your acupressure routine two or three times a day. It often takes at least four to six months of regular practice to see substantial pain relief for prolonged periods of time, so be patient.

Tips for Treatment

- Wash your hands and make sure they are clean and warm before touching yourself or someone else.
- Keep your fingernails short to avoid scratching or poking the skin.
- Keep it smooth: Apply gradual, steady pressure; hold; then gradually release the pressure. Avoid sharp pokes or jabs.
- Don't overdo. Every acupressure point requires a different amount of pressure. Some tender spots need only a gentle touch, whereas other points respond best to intense, steady pressure. In general the face, calves, and genitals should be handled gently; the neck, back, and buttocks can tolerate considerably more pressure.
- Remember, acupressure should not hurt. If a particular point feels uncomfortable when pressed, then gradually release the pressure until the pain subsides.
- Even if they are key points, don't apply pressure to areas of your body that have been burned, bruised, cut, sprained, or infected. Instead apply pressure to the points close to the injury to stimulate blood flow to the area.
- Apply warmth to the joints before beginning your acupressure session to relax stiff muscles and speed healing. Soaking in a hot bath or applying heat with a hot-water bottle or electric heating pad may help soothe and relax the muscles and joints, which will promote healing.

Top Twelve Acupressure Points for Arthritis

Hundreds of acupressure points exist on the body, but the following key points have proven particularly effective in managing arthritis pain.

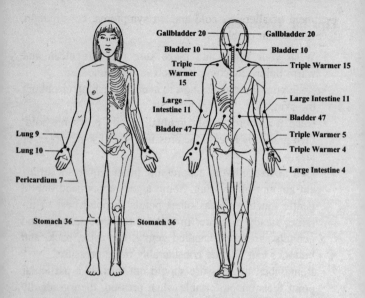

"Active Pond" (Triple Warmer 4)

LOCATION: Follow the outside of the arm to the hollow in the center of the wrist case.

BENEFITS: Relieves wrist, forearm, and elbow pain; reduces wrist inflammation and improves wrist flexibility. Also good for treatment of carpal tunnel syndrome and fever.

"Big Mound" (Pericardium 7)

LOCATION: In the middle of the inside wrist crease.

BENEFITS: Relieves pain in the palms of the hands and the middle fingers. Also good for treatment of appetite imbalance.

"Crooked Pond" (Large Intestine 11)

LOCATION: At the outer edge of the elbow crease.

BENEFITS: Reduces inflammation in the elbows and shoulders and eases pain in the arms and shoulders. Also good for treatment of allergies, cold and flu symptoms, constipation, fever, and skin problems.

"Fish Border" *(Lung 10)*

LOCATION: On the palm side of the hand in the center of the pad at the base of the thumb.

BENEFITS: Relieves pain in the hands. Also good for treatment of asthma, coughing, sore throat, and upset stomach.

"Gates of Consciousness" *(Gallbladder 20)*

LOCATION: Just below the base of the skull, in the hollow between the two large neck muscles, 2 to 3 inches apart, depending on the size of the head.

BENEFITS: Relieves arthritic pain throughout the body. Also good for treatment of back pain, dizziness, headaches, insomnia, and stiff neck.

"Great Abyss" *(Lung 9)*

LOCATION: In the hollow on the inside wrist crease just below the base of the thumb.

BENEFITS: Relieves wrist and arm pain. Also good for treatment of asthma, anxiety, coughing, and insomnia.

"Heavenly Pillar" *(Bladder 10)*

LOCATION: On the upper neck, ½ inch below the base of the skull on the ropy muscles ½ inch outward from either side of the spine.

BENEFITS: Relieves neck and back pain. Also good for treatment of anxiety and stress.

"Heavenly Rejuvenation" *(Triple Warmer 15)*

LOCATION: First locate the spot on the shoulders midway between the base of the neck and the outside of the shoulders. The correct position is ½ inch below this point.

BENEFITS: Relieves shoulder and neck pain. Also good for treatment of anxiety and for cold and flu symptoms.

"Joining the Valley" (Large Intestine 4)

LOCATION: On the outside of the hand, in the webbing between the thumb and index fingers at the highest spot of the muscle when the thumb and index fingers are brought close together.
BENEFITS: Reduces inflammation and eases arthritis pain throughout the body, especially in the hands, wrists, elbows, and shoulders. Also good for treatment of constipation, neck pain, headaches, and toothaches.

"Outer Gate" (Triple Warmer 5)

LOCATION: Flex the hand backward to find the wrist crease. The point is on the outside of the forearm, two finger widths down from the wrist crease, between the forearm bones.
BENEFITS: Relaxes and eases pain in the shoulders. Also good for treatment of anxiety and cold and flu symptoms.

"Sea of Vitality" (Bladder 47)

LOCATION: In the lower back, between the second and third lumbar vertebrae, two to four finger widths away from the spine at waist level.
BENEFITS: Relieves lower backache. Also good for treatment of fatigue and urinary problems.

"Three Mile Point" (Stomach 36)

LOCATION: Four finger widths below the kneecap and one finger width outside of the shinbone.
BENEFITS: Relieves arthritis pain throughout the body, especially in the knees. This point is known to renew energy and improve endurance. Also good for treatment of constipation, gas, nausea, and vomiting.

RESOURCES: ACUPRESSURE

Acupuncture and acupressure professionals must meet state-licensing or certification requirements in twenty-seven states and the District of Columbia.

For additional information on acupuncture and acupressure, as well as for free referrals to several practitioners in your area, contact:

The American Association for Acupuncture and Oriental Medicine
433 Front Street
Catasauqoa, Pennsylvania 18032-2506
(610) 433-2448

The Association publishes a monthly journal, *The American Acupuncturist.*

Acupressure Institute
1533 Shattuck Avenue
Berkeley, California 94709
(800) 442-2232
(415) 845-1059 in California

The Institute also publishes a catalog of publications, videos, and products involving acupressure and shiatsu therapy.

To confirm certification of a particular acupuncture or acupressure practitioner, contact:

The National Commission for the Certification of Acupuncturists
P.O. Box 97075
Washington, DC 20090
(202) 232-1404

CHAPTER EIGHT

Homeopathy: When Less Is More

Times are changing. A generation ago, Americans favored the high-tech approach to healing, but recently a growing number of people have turned to low-tech natural treatments for common medical problems, including arthritis. Though out of favor for some time, the two-hundred-year-old practice of homeopathy is an increasingly popular option for many Americans.

Homeopathy uses infinitesimal amounts of substances—plants, minerals, chemicals, and animal materials—to bolster the body's defensive mechanisms. The practice is based on a concept known as the Law of Similars, or "Like cures like." According to the theory, illnesses can be cured by giving the sick person tiny doses of a substance that would produce the symptoms of the disease in a healthy person if ingested in "material doses." The idea is akin to that of immunology, but the dosage is too small to trigger an immunological response. In fact the word *homeopathy* has its roots in the Greek words *homo,* meaning "like, similar" and *pathos,* meaning "suffering or disease."

For example homeopaths use belladonna, an extract from

the poisonous plant deadly nightshade, to treat fever and flu because at higher doses belladonna would cause a healthy person to experience fever and flulike symptoms. Keep in mind that the actual amount of belladonna is dramatically diluted in the homeopathic remedy. In fact many homeopathic remedies are diluted to such a degree that not a single molecule of the active ingredient can be found in the solution.

The reliance on dilution reflects the homeopathic Law of Infinitesimals; this theory states that the smaller the dose of active ingredient, the more effective the cure. However, for the process to work, each time the solution is diluted, it must be "potentized" (shaken) to create a "spiritlike" essence or "memory of the energy," which cures the body by activating its "vital force."

These homeopathic theories may seem contrary to common sense and the laws of physical science, but a number of studies published in respected medical journals show that homeopathic remedies work. For example in 1991 the *British Medical Journal* published an analysis of 105 clinical studies involving the efficacy of homeopathy, and 81 of them found that the homeopathic treatment was more effective than a placebo. Critics of homeopathy charged that many of the studies were poorly done, but a review of 26 of the better-controlled studies found that 15 studies demonstrated the benefit of homeopathic treatments.

And the evidence continues to mount. A 1994 study published in the British journal *The Lancet* found that homeopathic treatments outperformed a placebo in bringing relief to twenty-eight patients allergic to dust mites. That same year the first article was published in a peer-reviewed medical journal in the United States. In May 1994 the journal *Pediatrics* reported that among eighty-one children in Nicaragua treated for diarrhea, those given a homeopathic treatment in addition to the standard oral rehydration therapy got well faster than those who got the standard treatment alone.

Despite the evidence, no one really understands exactly how homeopathy works. Some experts have suggested that the medical enigma works because the repeated diluting and shaking of the substances creates a distinctive electrochemical pattern in the water. When a patient takes the homeopathic remedy, the electrochemical pattern in the solution is transferred and changes the electrochemical pattern of the water elsewhere in the body. Another theory argues that the "potentization" process somehow subtly changes the electromagnetic fields in the body. Both of these theories are difficult to understand—and to prove—because they involve energy changes at a subatomic level.

Still, one fascinating study has shown that homeopathic remedies are actually physically distinct from one another and from placebos. In 1983 scientists used nuclear magnetic resonance machines to measure the spin on subatomic particles in twenty-three homeopathic remedies. Each of the homeopathic remedies they tested had a distinct reading, but the placebo did not. Homeopathic remedies are distinctive, even if scientists cannot explain exactly why.

In the future, researchers will certainly explore various theories about homeopathy, trying to either prove or disprove its effectiveness. In the meantime you may want to consider adding homeopathic treatments to your arsenal of arthritis-fighting tools.

History of Homeopathy

In the early nineteenth century, Dr. Samuel Hahnemann (1755–1843), a German physician who had been trained in conventional medicine, developed the practice of homeopathy. During Hahnemann's day medical doctors commonly employed crude and often harmful practices, such as blood-letting and the use of massive doses of poorly understood drugs. One of the reasons Hahnemann developed the gentle practice of homeopathy was to counteract the harsh and often vulgar world of orthodox medicine in the 1800s.

Long before it become fashionable, Hahnemann believed that nutrition and exercise could help heal the human body. He tested other methods of treatment, often conducting experiments on himself. In an early experiment Hahnemann tested cinchona (also known as Peruvian bark), which is the natural source of quinine. When he ingested small doses of the bark, Hahnemann came down with fever, chills, thirst, and a pounding headache—the symptoms of malaria. He based his Law of Similars on his observation that the effectiveness of cinchona in treating malaria was linked to its ability to produce similar symptoms to those of the disease.

In further experiments Hahnemann learned that higher concentrations of substances caused more side effects but that he could dilute a medication and still preserve its healing powers through what he called the pharmacological process of "potentization." Hahnemann found that by repeatedly diluting a substance with distilled water or alcohol and shaking it vigorously between each dilution, he could increase the potency of the medicine. These findings resulted in Hahnemann's theory, the Law of Infinitesimals.

Homeopathy was put to the test in dealing with epidemic diseases, such as cholera, typhoid, yellow fever, and scarlet fever. The success of the treatment led to widespread interest in the practice of homeopathy. The first homeopathic college opened in Philadelphia in 1836, and eight years later a group of homeopaths formed the American Institute of Homeopathy, the first national medical organization in the country. By the end of the nineteenth century there were fifteen thousand homeopaths and twenty-two schools of homeopathy nationwide. Homeopathy also flourished and continues to thrive in Europe, particularly in Great Britain, where the queen of

England has her own homeopathic physician and the British National Health Service covers homeopathic procedures.

In the United States, however, homeopathy rapidly fell out of favor. At the end of the nineteenth century one out of every five American doctors practiced homeopathy, but by the middle of the twentieth century the American practice of homeopathy had all but died out. One reason was that the American Medical Association prohibited physicians who practiced homeopathy from joining their group and prohibited members from consulting with homeopaths. Another factor was that the discovery of antibiotics and other advances in modern medicine lured people to support a more "scientific" approach to healing.

Treat the Person, Not the Disease

Homeopaths and conventional doctors approach healing from different points of view. Homeopaths believe illness is not localized in one organ or manifested in one symptom, so when prescribing treatment they consider the entire person, both mind and body. Practitioners of conventional medicine, on the other hand, tend to focus on suppressing symptoms, taking little or no account of the person's emotional or overall physical condition.

Homeopaths consider physical symptoms positive signs that the body is hard at work defending and healing itself. Rather than trying to eliminate symptoms, homeopathic remedies sometimes even aggravate symptoms for a time as they stimulate the body's self-healing mechanism. The treatment is not intended for use with physical deformities, tissue damage, cancer, and situations when major surgery is indicated. But because the approach treats the person rather than a specific disease, there is no single treatment for arthritis, but instead a number of possible treatments, depending on the specific situation and symptoms.

Because homeopaths prescribe treatments based on a variety of very specific factors, the home use of homeopathic remedies should be limited to treatment of relatively minor ailments. If you experience recurrent or potentially dangerous symptoms, consider consulting with a trained homeopath.

A visit to a classical homeopath usually starts out with a long interview, including detailed questions about your medical history, as well as information on your overall energy, sensitivity to temperature and water, sleep habits, food preferences, and emotional state. All of these factors must be taken into account by a homeopath when deciding which of the more than two thousand remedies to prescribe.

Practicing Homeopathy

Unlike other medical practices, the selection of the appropriate homeopathic remedy varies from patient to patient, depending on the mental and emotional profile of the patient and the specific symptoms that are present. For example two people might pass a cold virus from one to the other, but each individual would receive different treatments, based on their specific conditions and temperament.

Homeopathic remedies are prepared according to standards of the *Homeopathic Pharmacopoeia of the United States;* they come in a variety of potencies, based on dilution. Homeopathic creams, ointments, and salves can be made by mixing diluted remedies with cream or gel base for topical use. The three most common forms of remedies are the mother tincture, *x*-potencies, and *c*-potencies.

- **The mother tincture.** The mother tincture is an alcohol-based extract of a specific substance. Mother tinctures are usually used topically.
- **X-potencies.** The *x* represents the Roman numeral 10,

and in homeopathic remedies with *x*-potencies the mother tincture has been diluted to one part in ten (one drop of tincture to every nine drops of alcohol). The number before the *x* tells how many times the mother tincture has been diluted. For example, a 12x potency represents 12 dilutions of one in ten. The more the substance is diluted, the more potent it becomes, so a remedy with a 30x potency is considered stronger or more potent than one with a 12x potency.

- *C*-potencies. The *c* represents the Roman numeral 100, so homeopathic remedies with a *c*-potency have been diluted to one part in one hundred (one drop of tincture to every ninety-nine drops of alcohol). Again, the number before the *c* represents the number of dilutions. A 3c potency represents a substance that has been diluted to one part in one hundred 3 times; by the time 3c is reached, the dilution is one part per million. In general, 6c is the potency recommended for most acute or self-limiting ailments, and 30c for chronic conditions or emergencies.

The 30c potency should not be administered for more than four doses without a clear and definite result. If your condition improves after four doses, wait and see what happens. If the symptoms return, take up to four more doses, then wait again. If you experience no improvement after four doses, discontinue the treatment and try something else or contact a qualified homeopath.

Homeopathic remedies come in pellet, tablet, and liquid form. The pellets and tablets consist primarily of sugar. Homeopathic tinctures contain relatively high levels of alcohol. When taking homeopathic pellets or tablets, avoid touching them. Instead shake the pellets into a spoon and place them under your tongue to allow them to dissolve.

* * *

WARNING: When you use the right remedy, it will work quickly and then you can discontinue treatment. Although negative reactions to homeopathic remedies are uncommon, they unquestionably occur and can be both unpleasant and long-lasting if the remedy that caused the reaction is repeated after the reaction has set in. If the local symptoms or your overall health get worse when taking a particular remedy, stop taking it. Wait for the aggravation to subside and then test it again. If the aggravation recurs, stop using the remedy and seek help from a professional homeopath.

Tips for Treatment

- Use a homeopathic remedy at least a half hour before or after eating or drinking coffee. Strong flavors can decrease the effectiveness of the remedies. Odors can also affect efficacy, so avoid strong smells, such as perfumes, chemical odors, and other scents.
- Know when to quit. If you give a treatment for a condition that clears up in fifteen minutes, you don't need to give another dose. If the symptom later returns, you can administer a second dose.

Homeopathic Treatments

Osteoarthritis

The following treatments can be used to deal with acute arthritis flare-ups associated with osteoarthritis:

- *Rhus tox. (Rhus toxicodendron)* 6c: Use if joint pain is worse first thing in the morning or after a period of rest, and gets better with continued motion. The pain is relieved by heat but made worse by damp, cold air. The pain becomes worse in the morning and after periods of rest, up with gradual movement. One dose four times a day for up to 2 weeks.

- *Bryonia (Bryonia alba or B. dioica)* 30c: Use for severe pain that feels worse with the slightest motion. The pain improves with cold and feels worse with heat treatment and movement. One dose three times a day for up to three doses. If the remedy works but the symptoms return after three doses, take up to three more doses, then wait again. If there is no improvement after three doses, try another remedy or consult a homeopath.

- *Pulsatilla (Pulsatilla nigricans)* 6c: Use when joint pain seems to wander from joint to joint on a day-to-day basis. The pain is made worse by heat and when you are feeling weepy. One dose four times a day for up to 2 weeks.

- *Calcarea phos. (Calcarea phosphorica)* 6c: Use when affected joints feel numb and cold; symptoms become worse during weather changes. One dose four times a day for up to 2 weeks.

- *Ledum (Ledum palustre)* 6c: Use when pain involves small joints, such as toes and fingers; the joints may crack and the pain may be relieved by cold treatment. One dose four times a day for up to 2 weeks.

- *Arnica (Arnica montana)* 30c: Use when joint pain is made worse by an injury. One dose three times a day for up to three doses. If the remedy works but the symptoms return after three doses, take up to three more doses, then wait again. If there is no improvement after three doses, try another remedy or consult a homeopath.

- *Aconite (Aconitum napellus)* 30c: Use for severe pain and flare-ups in cold weather. One dose three times a day for up to three doses. If the remedy works but the symptoms return after three doses, take up to three more doses, then wait again. If there is no improvement after three doses, try another remedy or consult a homeopath.

Rheumatoid Arthritis

Rheumatoid arthritis is an autoimmune disease that in severe cases can cause bone deformity. The following treatments can be used to deal with pain associated with rheumatoid arthritis:

- *Aesculus (Aesculus hippocastanum)* 6c: Use for pain around sacroiliac joint; pain is worse after walking or bending over. One dose three times a day for up to 5 days.
- *Belladonna (Atropha belladonna)* 30c: Use for shooting pain or achiness in the legs strong enough to cause limping. One dose every 2 hours for up to three doses. If the remedy works but the symptoms return after three doses, take up to three more doses, then wait again. If there is no improvement after three doses, try another remedy or consult a homeopath.
- *Rhododendron (Rhododendron chrysanthum)* 6c: Use when the pain is worse before rain or a storm. The pain often feels worse in hot weather. One dose every 2 hours for up to 2 days.
- *Rhus tox. (Rhus toxicodendron)* 6c: Use for pain that is worse in the morning and after periods of rest and feels better after use. One dose three times a day for up to 3 days.
- *Dulcamara (Solanum dulcamara)* 6c: Use for neck pain similar to that of a stiff neck caused by resting in an awkward position. Pain relieved by heat, aggravated by chill. One dose every 4 hours for 2 days.
- *Bryonia (Bryonia alba or B. dioica)* 6c: Use for neck pain that feels worse with movement. The pain feels much worse with the slightest motion. One dose every 4 hours for up to 2 days.
- *Causticum (Causticum hahnemanni)* 6c: Use for pain at the nape of the neck accompanied by soreness between

the shoulder blades. One dose every 4 hours for up to 2 days.

- *Ferrum (Ferrum metallicum)* 6c: Use for shoulder pain that improves with walking; pain worse at night and with cold. One dose four times day for up to 2 weeks.

- *Benzoic ac. (Benzoicum acidum)* 6c: Use for swollen and painful knees, when the arthritis causes a cracking sound. One dose every 2 hours for up to 3 days.

- *Berberis (Berberis vulgaris)* 6c: Use for stiff, sore knees. One dose every 2 hours for up to 3 days.

- *Caulophyllum (Caulophyllum thalictroides)* 30c: Use for arthritic pain in the ankles and toes. One dose every 4 hours for up to three doses. If the remedy works but the symptoms return after three doses, take up to three more doses, then wait again. If there is no improvement after three doses, try another remedy or consult a homeopath.

Gout

Gout responds well to traditional drug and dietary treatment. However, the following homeopathic treatments may help during a gout attack:

- *Colchicum (Colchicum autumnale)* 6c: Use when the affected joint is excruciatingly painful and the person feels weak and nauseated. One dose every 15 minutes for up to 3 hours.

- *Arnica (Arnica montana)* 30c: Use when the gout-affected joint feels bruised. One dose every 15 minutes for up to three doses. If the remedy works but the symptoms return after three doses, take up to three more doses, then wait again. If there is no improvement after three doses, try another remedy or consult a homeopath.

- *Ledum (Ledum palustre)* 6c: Use when joints are swollen and feel cold; the pain eases with cold treatment and grows worse with movement. One dose every 15 minutes for up to 3 hours.

- *Urtica (Urtica urens)* 30c: Use when the affected joints itch and burn. One dose every 15 minutes for up to three doses. If the remedy works but the symptoms return after three doses, take up to three more doses, then wait again. If there is no improvement after three doses, try another remedy or consult a homeopath.

Infective Arthritis

This rare form of arthritis is caused by a bacterial infection that invades the joints. Prompt medical attention is necessary; antibiotics are needed to cure the infection. The following homeopathic remedies can provide some relief *while you seek appropriate medical care:*

- *Aconite (Aconitum napellus)* 30c: Use when the infection comes on suddenly, accompanied by high fever. One dose every hour for up to three doses. If the remedy works but the symptoms return after three doses, take up to three more doses, then wait again. If there is no improvement after three doses, try another remedy or consult a homeopath.
- *Bryonia (Bryonia alba or B. dioica)* 30c: Use when the affected joint is swollen, painful, and sensitive to touch. The pain will feel significantly worse with the slightest motion. One dose every hour for up to three doses. If the remedy works but the symptoms return after three doses, take up to three more doses, then wait again. If there is no improvement after three doses, try another remedy or consult a homeopath.
- *Belladonna (Atropha belladonna)* 30c: Use when severe, sudden joint pain is accompanied by high fever and delirium. Any movement causes severe pain. One dose ev-

ery hour for up to three doses. If the remedy works but
the symptoms return after three doses, take up to three
more doses, then wait again. If there is no improvement
after three doses, try another remedy or consult a homeopath.

RESOURCES: HOMEOPATHY

Homeopathy is practiced by medical doctors (M.D.'s), osteopaths (D.O.'s), naturopaths (N.D.'s), chiropractors (D.C.'s),
and dentists (D.D.S.'s). Some states also allow chiropractors,
family nurse practitioners, acupuncturists, and physician as-
sistants to obtain licensure.

For an information packet of homeopathy and a directory
of practitioners, contact:

The National Center for Homeopathy
801 North Fairfax Street, Suite 306
Alexandria, Virginia 22314
(703) 548-7790

There is a $6 fee for the information packet and
directory. The Center also publishes the monthly
magazine *Homeopathy Today,* as well as other books and
products.

The International Foundation for Homeopathy
P.O. Box 7
Edmons, Washington 98020
(206) 776-4147

There is a $4 fee for the information packet and
directory.

Manufacturers of homeopathic medicines that offer mail-
order catalogs include the following:

The Apothecary
5415 Cedar Lane
Bethesda, Maryland 20814
(301) 530-0800

Apthorp Pharmacy
2201 Broadway at 78th Street
New York, New York 10024
(800) 775-3582
(212) 877-3480

Bailey's Pharmacy
175 Harvard Avenue
Allston, Massachusetts 02134
(800) 239-6206
(617) 782-7202

Boericke and Tafel, Inc.
2381 Circadian Way
Santa Rosa, California 95407
(707) 571-8202

Budget Pharmacy
3001 N.W. 7th Street
Miami, Florida 33125
(800) 221-9772

Dolisos America, Inc.
3014 Rigel Avenue
Las Vegas, Nevada 89102
(702) 871-7153

Five Elements Center
115 Route 46W
Building D, Suite 29
Mount Lakes, New Jersey 07046
(201) 402-8510

Hahnemann Pharmacy
828 San Pablo Avenue
Albany, California 94706
(510) 527-3003

Homeopathic Educational Services
2124 Kittredge Street
Berkeley, California 94707
(510) 649-0294

Homeopathy Overnight
4111 Simon Road
Youngstown, Ohio 44512
(800) ARNICA-30

Humphreys Pharmacal Inc.
63 Meadow Road
Rutherford, New Jersey 07070
(201) 933-7744

Luyties Pharmaceutical Co.
4200 Laclede Avenue
St. Louis, Missouri 63108
(800) 325-8080

Santa Monica Homeopathic Co.
629 Broadway
Santa Monica, California 90401
(310) 395-1131

Standard Homeopathy Co.
P.O. Box 61067
154 W. 131st Street
Los Angeles, California 90061
(213) 321-4284

Taylor's Pharmacy
230 North Park Avenue
Winter Park, Florida 32789
(407) 644-1025

Washington Homeopathic Pharmacy
4914 Del Ray Avenue
Bethesda, Maryland 20814
(301) 656-1695

Weleda Pharmacy, Inc.
175 North Route 9W
Congers, New York 10920
(914) 268-8572

CHAPTER NINE

Just Imagine: Healing Using the Mind-Body Connection

Arthritis expresses itself in the form of joint stiffness and pain, but your state of mind can go a long way toward making your condition better—or worse. What you think and feel affects your experience of pain. That's not to say that the pain is "all in your head," but rather that you can use your mind to help minimize the pain and make it more manageable.

Consider the impact of stress on arthritis. Most arthritis sufferers can testify that a long and stressful day can lead to tight muscles, which squeeze and apply pressure on the joints and exacerbate pain, in addition to bringing on that frazzled and worn-out feeling.

So relax.

Though easier said than done, relaxation can noticeably relieve arthritis pain, sometimes in a matter of minutes. Remember, stress reduction doesn't have to come out of a bottle. By learning and practicing techniques of stress reduction and relaxation, you can make significant strides toward managing your arthritis pain.

How Your Body Reacts to Stress

Life is stressful. To your body, stress is any challenge or change you confront. An auto accident is stressful, and so is buying a new car. Losing an important contest or missing out on a promotion is stressful, and so is winning or getting a promotion, no matter how well deserved. A divorce is stressful, and so is falling in love. And as arthritis sufferers are well aware, living with chronic pain is stressful in a number of ways.

To be alive is to experience stress. The secret of course is learning how to control stress and respond to it in a way that prevents it from taking an undue toll on your physical and psychological well-being.

Our understanding of how the body reacts to stress can be traced back to Walter B. Cannon, a physiologist at Harvard University at the turn of the century. Cannon first recognized and defined the so-called fight-or-flight response to stress, which involves a number of biochemical changes that happen to the body in preparation for dealing with danger. This response made sense in evolutionary terms: Early man needed quick bursts of energy to escape danger or fight off life-threatening predators. Though modern man faces fewer of these life-or-death threats, our bodies still respond to stressful events in much the same way as our prehistoric relatives.

In the body any stressor (either real or imagined) causes the cerebral cortex of the brain to trigger an alarm to the hypothalamus in the midbrain. The hypothalamus then charges into action, sending messages throughout the body to prepare for an emergency. As a result your heart rate increases, your breathing grows faster, your muscles tense, your metabolism kicks into high gear, and your blood pressure soars. Your blood concentrates in your muscles, leaving your hands and feet cold and your stomach filled with butterflies. Your hearing becomes more acute and your pupils dilate. You're ready to deal with anything.

During this stress response your body also releases adrenaline, epinephrine, and other chemicals that inhibit the immune system in addition to interfering with digestion, reproduction, growth, and tissue repair. These stress responses can cause serious health problems if stress continues for long periods of time.

Fortunately it is relatively easy for the body to flip a switch and reverse the stress response. Your body begins to relax as soon as your brain receives the signal that the danger has passed and it's safe to relax. The brain cancels the emergency signals to the central nervous system, and within about three minutes the panic messages cease and relaxation begins. The heart rate and breathing slow, and the other systems return to their normal levels.

Your brain can't tell whether the relaxation response was triggered by a change in circumstances or a change in your attitude. Either way the relaxation is the same. Just as chronic, prolonged stress can make arthritis pain more intense, so reversing that stress can help to ease the pain and promote relaxation.

PHYSICAL SYMPTOMS OF STRESS

- Anger and irritability
- Backaches
- Constipation
- Depression
- Diarrhea
- Elevated blood pressure
- Fatigue
- Headaches and migraines
- Indigestion
- Insomnia and sleep irregularities
- Irritable bowel syndrome
- Muscle spasms
- Muscle tension
- Neckaches
- Obesity
- Tics and twitches
- Ulcers
- Weakness

You Can Change Your Perception of Pain

Most people are controlled by their pain. They surrender to it—or they use medication to dull the pain. But there are concrete steps you can take to understand your pain and take charge of it.

Pain experts believe that pain has both physical and psychological origins. When face-to-face with the same level and type of pain, some people tough it out and others give up because they have lower pain thresholds or tolerances.

Pain can be divided into four basic categories: first, the initial sensation (when you first experience a feeling); second, when the sensation turns to pain; third, when pain becomes intolerable; and finally when you cannot withstand the pain, even with external encouragement (this is the upper threshold of tolerance). Researchers have found that people can learn to tolerate higher levels of pain when encouraged and trained. How you feel about pain can actually change the way you perceive it.

As part of learning to control your pain, you can learn techniques for reducing anxiety by taking time for mental calming and the release of daily stress. The following self-help techniques can be very helpful in minimizing muscle tension and promoting relaxation.

Biofeedback

Biofeedback involves training yourself to use your mind to voluntarily control the body's internal systems. The key to biofeedback is practice, so that you can learn the precise effect of mind over body. To learn the skill, you attach electrodes to various part of your body to measure your heart rate, blood pressure, temperature, muscle tension, and brain wave pattern. A small machine on the other end of the wires displays the data, usually in the form of pictures, graphic lines, or audible beeps. You can literally watch yourself relax or grow more tense.

To learn to relax, patients learn to produce alpha brain wave patterns. In this case the electrodes attach to an electroencephalograph, which displays the brain waves on an oscilloscope. When alpha waves are present, the machine sounds a tone. The patient's quest is to sustain the tone by holding on to the thought or visualization that proves soothing and relaxing. Most people can learn to produce alpha brain waves in a few training sessions with a biofeedback clinician.

By carefully studying the measurable changes in your

body as you relax and change your thought patterns, you can actually learn to slow yourself down and actually control your body's internal processes. This training in mind over matter can be very useful in learning to relax. Most of us have no trouble learning how to be stressed out, but it takes long hours of practice to learn to physiologically slow down—but it can be done.

The goal of course is to become so familiar with the sensations associated with a particular physical state that you can control your body without being hooked up to the machine. Biofeedback by itself does nothing to control arthritis pain, but the relaxation that it brings can go a long way toward easing your aching joints. The technique is particularly effective in the treatment of chronic pain and stress-related disorders.

If you'd like to try biofeedback, ask your physician for a referral to an outpatient pain clinic or look for biofeedback centers listed in the phone book. Before making an appointment, ask about fees and whether or not the service would be covered by your health insurance plan.

For a referral to someone qualified to teach you the techniques of biofeedback, contact: The Association for Applied Psychophysiology and Biofeedback, 10200 West 44th Avenue, Suite 304, Wheat Ridge, Colorado 80033; (303) 422-8436.

Breathing

Most people take their breathing for granted. But breathing is actually a complex process involving the transfer of oxygen to the tissues and the removal of the waste product carbon dioxide.

When people are under stress or in pain, they often breathe poorly, taking shallow, weak breaths. With an inadequate supply of oxygen (and the inadequate removal of waste products), the body is less able to manage stress, resulting in anxiety, panic attacks, depression, headaches, fatigue, and muscle tension. On the other hand healthful, deep breathing helps to relax the body and quiet the mind. Good breathing techniques can be practiced separately or along with other relaxation exercises.

Consider what happens inside your body when you draw a breath: The air is pulled in through your nose, where the nasal passages warm it to body temperature, filter out foreign particles, and add a touch of humidity to keep the lungs moist. In the lungs the air travels along a series of tubes or branches to tiny air sacs called alveoli, which inflate when air fills the lungs and contract when air is exhaled. Blood vessels and capillaries next to the alveoli absorb the oxygen and pass it on to the heart. In the heart the oxygenated blood is pumped out and distributed throughout the body. The blood cells then trade fresh oxygen for carbon dioxide, which returns to the heart and works its way back through the capillaries to the alveoli, through the lungs, and out of the body as you exhale.

The process of respiration is the same whether you use chest breathing (also called thoracic breathing) or abdominal breathing (also called diaphragmatic breathing). However, abdominal breathing is much more efficient and relaxing.

When people are nervous or stressed, they usually engage in chest breathing, which tends to be shallow, rapid, and irregular, involving only the top part of the lungs. When a chest-breather draws in the air, the chest expands and the shoulders rise, but the air does not entirely fill the lungs. This results in inadequate oxygenation of the blood, which causes the heart rate to increase and stress to build.

Abdominal breathing is the natural pattern for newborn babies and sleeping adults, but most adults don't do it during their waking hours. To properly nourish and oxygenate the lungs, air should be drawn deeply into the lungs, allowing the chest to fill entirely with air and the belly to rise and fall slowly. Breathing should be even and unconstricted.

When you become aware of your breathing, you will inhale more fully and feel the muscle tension and stress melt away. You will experience a greater sense of calm and well-being almost immediately as you feel the improved oxygenation in your tissues.

Go ahead and take a deep breath. Fill your lungs with air, then slowly exhale. Do it again. Put one hand on your abdomen and the other on the center of your chest. Without attempting to change your breathing pattern, take note of how you are breathing. Then move on to concentrated, deep abdominal breathing. Yoga (discussed on page 166) focuses on deep breathing, in addition to stretching exercises.

Whenever you practice deep breathing, if you experience shortness of breath, heart palpitations, or a feeling that you can't get enough air, stop immediately and return to your regular breathing pattern.

Controlling Your Emotions

When diagnosed with arthritis or any other chronic disease, many people feel depressed, stressed, and angry. These emotions can cause anxiety and frustration, which in turn can make matters worse by causing you to tighten the muscles around your joints. Arthritis is not caused by emotional stress, but emotional turmoil can make symptoms flare. And conversely emotional balance and release of stress can sometimes put symptoms into remission.

It can be difficult—or impossible—to relax and minimize the daily stress of living with a chronic health problem until you own up to the emotional issues behind the illness. Arthritis can be a particularly difficult disease to deal with because of its cyclic nature and unknown origins.

Depression is a normal and common response to living with arthritis. It is difficult to accept limitations on what you can and cannot do. The disease can change the familiar patterns of your life and make you feel you have little or no control over your life. The pain, concern about medical expenses, and apprehension about your future health can compound the stress and depression. In addition some arthritis medications can cause depression as a side effect.

In situations when a medical professional recommends bed rest, some families experience stress because the distribution of work and support has changed. It is always best to discuss these issues openly rather than wait and allow resentments to build up. In families that find frank discussions difficult, a professional family counselor may be able to help the entire family accept the situation and work on solutions that meet the needs of all family members.

Many people can resolve their feelings by talking things over with a loved one, a friend, or a professional counselor. Others find it helpful to participate in a support group for people with arthritis. These groups can be a tremendous source of encouragement and support. Support groups known as arthritis clubs are located nationwide; for information contact the local chapter of the Arthritis Foundation listed in your telephone directory. Other groups may be offered through the social service department of your local hospital.

Another option is cognitive behavior therapy, which teaches a variety of coping skills to help people control the thoughts, feelings, and actions that affect the pain. Some of the techniques involved repeating the word *relax* with deep breathing before activities that often bring on pain.

For a referral to a cognitive behavioral therapist who specializes in pain control, contact the Association for Advancement of Behavior Therapy, 305 Seventh Avenue, New York,

New York 10001; (212) 647-1890. There is a $5 fee for an information packet and list of qualified therapists in your area.

Hypnosis

Hypnosis can be used to help you relax and control your response to pain, including pain associated with arthritis. In fact some experts consider the method more effective and longer-lasting than acupuncture or aspirin, and it's free of side effects.

First get over the horror-movie image of the evil hypnotist putting the unwitting patient into a sleepy-eyed trance. In truth, during hypnosis the participant is in a highly alert state, deeply concentrating on the suggestions of the hypnotist. In most hypnosis sessions you would start by closing your eyes and thinking relaxing thoughts. The hypnotist would then guide you into deeper states of relaxation and focused concentration. At this point you are well aware of everything going on around you, but you are also more open to the power of suggestion. In such a state you may be more responsive to suggestions of new ways to interpret the pain signals associated with arthritis. For example some people who have been successfully hypnotized have been able to change the feeling of pain into a tingly or numb sensation by changing their thought patterns about the pain.

Of course hypnosis doesn't always work; some people are more responsive to the approach than others. But it is estimated that at least half of the people who try hypnosis find full or partial pain relief after several sessions.

If you want to consider pain management through hypnosis, ask your doctor for a referral to a psychiatrist or therapist qualified in the field. Don't just look in the phone book; many states have no licensing requirements for hypnotists. If your doctor can't make a referral, consider contacting one of the following professional organizations:

Academy of Scientific Hypnotherapy
P.O. Box 12041
San Diego, California 92112
(619) 427-6225

American Council of Hypnotist Examiners
1147 East Broadway, Suite 340
Glendale, California 91205
(818) 242-1159

American Hypnosis Association
18607 Ventura Boulevard, Suite 310
Tarzana, California 91356
(818) 344-4464

American Institute of Hypnotherapy
16842 Von Karman Avenue
#475
Irvine, California 92714
(800) 872-9996

American Society of Clinical Hypnosis
2200 East Devon Avenue, Suite 291
Des Plaines, Illinois 60018
(708) 297-3317

National Guild of Hypnotists
P.O. Box 308
Merrimack, New Hampshire 03054-0308
(603) 429-9438

Society for Clinical and Experimental Hypnosis
3905 Vincennes Road
Indianapolis, Indiana 46268
(317) 228-8073

Massage

Massage can be a very effective way of reducing stress. The technique, which involves soothing touch of the muscles, soft tissues, and ligaments of the body, helps to stimulate blood circulation and lower blood pressure.

There are two main types of massage: shiatsu and Swedish. Shiatsu involves finger pressure at key points on the body, very much like acupressure. The technique was developed in Japan at roughly the same time as acupressure was being refined in China.

Swedish massage includes four distinctive types of movements, each including continual, rhythmic motions and constant contact with the body. The techniques include

- *Effleurage:* This touch involves rhythmic, soothing strokes with open hands, the heels, the palms, or the thumbs. In some cases massage oil or cream is used to make motions smooth and even.
- *Percussion:* This technique includes brisk motions with alternate hands, such as chopping, pummeling, clapping, or tapping. It stimulates the skin and promotes circulation.
- *Petrissage:* This type of touch includes kneading, rolling, squeezing, lifting, and pressing the skin to stretch and stimulate the muscles. One hand should release its grip when the other takes over.
- *Pressure:* This technique involves the focused pressure, using small circular movements made with the thumbs, fingertips, or heel of the hand. It should be used at local tension spots or knotted muscles. The pressure should be held for about ten seconds, followed by effleurage to soothe the area.

Swedish massage can be used to diminish arthritis pain by affecting the mind and nervous system. Just as with gate-control theory in acupressure, the nervous system can process only a limited amount of sensory information. When the nervous system is overloaded, certain parts of it effectively shut down. For example if you're feeling excruciating arthritis pain in your right hand, you may be able to short-circuit that pain message to the brain by deeply massaging the forearms and shoulders.

Three recent studies on children with arthritis, asthma, and diabetes suggest that short daily massage significantly diminishes the symptoms of the various illnesses. Researchers at University of Miami School of Medicine found that when parents gave their children a fifteen- to twenty-minute massage every night, the children experienced significantly less pain.

When using massage to combat arthritis pain, stimulate the muscles attached to the tendons leading to the painful joints. For example for arthritis in the ankle or foot, massage the calf and shin area. (For more information on pressure points, see the chapter on acupressure.)

For more information on therapeutic massage, contact:

American Massage Therapy Association
820 Davis Street, Suite 100
Evanston, Illinois 60201
(708) 864-0123

American Oriental Bodywork Therapy Association
Glendale Executive Campus
1000 White Horse Road
Vorhees, New York 08043
(609) 782-1616

Associated Bodywork and Massage Professionals
28677 Buffalo Park Road

Evergreen, Colorado 80439-7347
(303) 674-8478

Meditation

Meditation comes in a variety of forms and traditions, but at the most basic level the practice involves attempting to focus your complete attention on one thing at a time. As most people discover when they try meditation, the mind tends to wander; it can be challenging to remain focused on a single object without distracting thoughts interfering with the concentration.

This back-and-forth struggle for control of the thoughts is not only natural, it can be therapeutic: It teaches the person meditating that there is a choice about what to think about and how to feel. Eventually it becomes clear that it is impossible to feel tense or angry or hostile when your mind is focused somewhere else. Meditation helps you relax because your mind no longer dwells on the negative stimulus since it is busy thinking about the target object.

Research has shown that meditation helps the body relax. For example back in 1968 researchers at Harvard Medical School found that when people practiced Transcendental Meditation (a type of mantra meditation), their heart rate and breathing slowed, their oxygen consumption dropped by 20 percent, their blood lactate levels dropped, their skin resistance to electrical current increased, and their brain wave patterns showed greater alpha wave activity—all physiological signs of deep relaxation.

To experiment with the technique of meditation, find a quiet place where you are not apt to be interrupted. Sit in a firm chair with your back as straight as possible. (You may prefer lying down flat on the ground, depending on the type of meditation you will be doing.)

There are three common forms of meditation, each with a different object of focus:

- *Mantra meditation* involves repeating (either aloud or silently) a word, syllable, or group of words. Each time you breathe out, you recite a neutral syllable (such as *ommmm*) or a soothing word (such as *peace* or *calm*) or a phrase (such as *it's okay*).
- *Gazing meditation* involves looking at an object such as a candle flame, a stone, or a flower to keep your attention focused. The object should be about one foot away from your face. Gaze at it rather than stare, keeping your eyes relaxed. Don't try to think about the object in words, just look at it without judgment.
- *Breathing meditation* involves focusing on the rising and falling of your breath. Some people consider this the most relaxing form of meditation. Draw a deep breath, focusing on the inhalation, the pause before you exhale, the exhalation, and the pause before you inhale again. When you exhale, say to yourself, "One." Each time you complete a breath and exhale, count again, one through four, then start over with one. The counting helps clear your mind of other thoughts.

With each type of meditation, start the session by inhaling deeply and pausing to enjoy the feeling of fullness. Then exhale fully, imagining that you are releasing all the tension in your body. During the time of meditation if thoughts about your daily life slip into your mind (and they almost certainly will, especially when you're first starting out), accept them and let them drift away without worry.

Try meditating for five to ten minutes at first, then work up to fifteen to twenty minutes once or twice a day. The more you practice, the better you'll get at freeing your mind of cluttering thoughts. At the end of the session you should feel much more relaxed and calm.

For more information on meditation, refer to books in the library or contact the Foundation for Human Understanding, P.O. Box 1009, Grants Pass, Oregon 97526; (503) 597-4360.

Pain Centers

In the past fifteen years or so, a growing number of medical centers have established special centers for the treatment of chronic pain, including the pain associated with arthritis. Those people who experience chronic pain often cannot work, rest well at night, or go through their daily routines without feeling exhausted. The pain can make the person feel depressed and cranky, which over the long haul can interfere with relationships with loved ones.

Pain centers, which are often affiliated with university hospitals or medical centers, often provide a range of services and techniques to help people learn to alleviate their pain or to cope with it. After diagnosing the source of pain, the doctors and specialists design a treatment plan that could include behavior modification, changes in lifestyle, as well as a number of the techniques described in this chapter.

For more information on pain centers and a list of accredited pain treatment programs, contact the Commission of Accreditation of Rehabilitation Facilities, 4891 East Grant Road, Tucson, Arizona 85715; (520) 325-1044.

Progressive Relaxation

Done properly, progressive relaxation can lead to profound calm, with the potential of temporary pain relief. Start by lying on your back on the floor, with your legs flat and your arms loose at your sides. Close your eyes and breathe deeply.

Once you are calm, you can begin systematically to tense

and relax every muscle in your body. Start with your feet: tense the muscles in your feet for thirty seconds or so, then relax, allowing your feet to feel heavy and relaxed. Then move on to your calves, thighs, abdomen, buttocks, hands, forearms, upper arms, shoulders, and face.

When you finish, your muscles should feel soothed and relaxed. Lie quietly and enjoy the feeling of complete relaxation.

This technique is helpful because most people do not realize which of their muscles are chronically tense. By working through the muscles in the body, the technique helps people identify particular muscles and muscle groups that tend to collect tension and stress.

Visualization

You can reduce stress with a tremendously powerful tool you always have at your disposal: your imagination. Through visualization you can ease the symptoms of stress by changing your thoughts. This practice builds on the idea that you are what you think you are. All your thoughts become reality. For example if you think anxious thoughts, you become tense; if you think sad thoughts, you become unhappy. On the other hand if you think soothing, positive thoughts, you will feel relaxed and have a more positive outlook.

Visualization can bring on a deep state of relaxation if you're willing and able to use your imagination creatively. Sit down in a comfortable position or lie on the floor in a quiet, dimly lit room. Tense all your muscles at once and hold for thirty seconds. Remember to breathe deeply as you contract your muscles. Then relax every muscle and allow all the tension to drain from your body. Continue to inhale and exhale slowly and fully.

Now that you have relaxed your muscles, you can begin the visualization part of the exercise. First concentrate on your breathing, feeling the regular rhythm of each breath. Clear your mind of all thoughts, then imagine that you are in a peaceful setting—walking along a sandy beach, lying in a meadow of wildflowers on a spring day, or looking out over an evergreen mountain range. Use all your senses: Smell the ocean mist, feel the warm sun caress your back. The more specific your fantasy, the more real it will seem. And the more real it seems, the more likely the arthritis pain will melt away, forgotten and unfelt.

At the end of the session, which should last about twenty minutes, gradually bring yourself back to "real time." When you open your eyes and get back to your daily routine, you will probably feel at ease, relaxed, and refreshed.

CHAPTER TEN

Hydrotherapy: Running Hot and Cold

Water can be very healing. Swimming can be excellent physical therapy; a whirlpool bath can soothe sore muscles; and warm compresses can increase blood circulation to certain tissues. The Greek god of medicine, Aesculapius, used bathing and massage to cure disease. Hippocrates also prescribed water cures, including drinking water to reduce fever.

Hydrotherapy—the use of water in the treatment of disease—recognizes that different temperatures of water have different effects on the body. If hot water is used, either in the form of a hot bath for the entire body or a hot compress for a localized site, the skin becomes red as blood is drawn to the surface. This warm blood then returns to the deeper blood vessels in the body, spreading the warmth. On the other hand cold water causes the blood vessels to contract, driving blood away from the surface of the skin. Often there is a secondary warming effect with cold treatments as the warmer blood from deeper in the body is pumped to the surface of the skin.

Cold water tends to be energizing. It can alleviate pain by acting as an anesthetic, in addition to lowering fever and reducing swelling caused by an injury. Hot water tends to be relaxing. Hot baths promote perspiration, which help to eliminate toxins from the body. Hot water increases blood flow and causes increased inflammation after an injury, but it can reduce pain and promote healing twenty-four hours after injury, when swelling is no longer of great concern.

In most cases hot-water treatments should be followed by brief cool or cold treatments to help restore the normal body temperature. Otherwise you could be at risk of dizziness or fainting, since in response to the heat the blood is drawn to the surface skin and away from the internal organs.

If your goal is to increase circulation, one of the most effective methods is to alternate between cold and hot treatments.

Hydrotherapy and Arthritis

Most arthritis sufferers can get temporary relief from arthritis pain by using hot or cold treatments. These treatments can be especially helpful before and after exercise.

Cool Down

Cold therapy (also called cryotherapy) includes the use of an ice pack (or a makeshift ice pack made of a bag of frozen vegetables or a wet towel placed in the freezer to chill for ten minutes or so).

The cold treatment often works better than heat for arthritis pain, especially pain and joint swelling associated with inflammation. The cold tends to penetrate farther and the pain relief often lasts longer than the results of heat treatment. More important, the cold also helps to reduce inflammation.

In addition to chronic pain, overuse injuries typically respond better to cold treatment. If you've overdone it and you're paying the price for your vigor, apply an ice pack to the affected area for fifteen to twenty minutes, then remove it for fifteen to twenty minutes. This on-again, off-again cycle can be repeated for hours if necessary.

Turn Up the Heat

Heat treatments promote relaxation and increase circulation in the affected area, resulting in temporary relief of pain and stiffness. However, heat treatments have a significant downside: They exacerbate inflammation.

Heat treatments (also called thermotherapy) can be applied as moist heat, using a bath, shower, or whirlpool to moisten and warm the skin. Dry heat requires the use of an electric heating pad or infrared heat lamp.

Following heat treatment, cool down using either a towel wrung out in cold water or a short, tepid shower. This facilitates your body's return to a normal temperature.

There are a number of different ways of applying heat treatments, including

- **A hot soak.** Many arthritis sufferers find relief after a relaxing soak in a warm tub for fifteen or twenty minutes. Hydrotherapy treats the whole body at once, allowing for the relaxation of many painful joints at one time. In addition the buoyancy of the water eases the strain on weight-bearing joints. A whirlpool can also add a gentle massaging action.
- **Hot-water scrub.** Consider a hot-water scrub to boost blood circulation throughout the body. Turn on the hot water and wet the middle part of a medium-size cotton towel. Wring out most of the water, then briskly rub yourself with the steamy hot towel. Systematically work across your entire body, until you feel warm and invigorated.
- **Hot wax.** Warm paraffin wax treatments can ease the pain in the fingers and feet. The hands or feet are dipped

several times in a thick mixture of melted paraffin and mineral oil until a wax coating forms. The area is then wrapped in plastic and covered with a moist towel to trap the heat. The wax is peeled away after fifteen or twenty minutes of deep heating.

- **Heat lamps.** The affected area is placed under an infrared bulb, which releases a controlled amount of heat. (This is not the same as ultraviolet light, which is used in sunlamps.) Heat-lamp treatment is often called diathermy.
- **Ultrasound.** Ultrasonic waves are directed at the affected area, where they penetrate the skin and cause warmth. (Other heat treatments merely heat the surface of the skin, relying on increased blood flow to provide the rest of the healing benefits.) While successful with some arthritis patients, this treatment is more commonly used with muscle injuries. The deep heating often works so quickly that the entire treatment lasts just two to ten minutes.

CAUTION: HOT! CAUTION: COLD!

- To avoid burns, never apply heat to one area for more than twenty to thirty minutes. To avoid freezing, never apply cold to an area for more than fifteen to twenty minutes. Of course remove the cold pack if the skin feels numb.
- Forgo heat or cold treatments if you have poor circulation, poor sensation, or cardiovascular problems. Instead use warm or cool treatments, not hot and cold.

Hot:	98–104 degrees F
Warm:	93–97 degrees F
Tepid:	81–92 degrees F
Cool:	66–80 degrees F
Cold:	55–65 degrees F

- Exercise caution when using heating pads and cold packs. Don't place the heat or cold source directly on the skin; use a towel between the device and your skin. Never lie on top of a heating pad; instead put the pad on top of the painful area.
- When using any form of heat or cold treatment, check your skin every five minutes for signs of excessive redness and burning or excessive whiteness and freezing.
- Avoid using hydrotherapy until at least an hour and a half after a meal. (The blood circulation will be needed for digestion.)
- Diabetics should avoid all heat treatments in their legs.

NOT JUST AN ORDINARY BATH

To enjoy additional therapeutic benefits, you can add herbs to your bath water. For best results run the bath water at about 96 degrees F. Soak in the tub for twenty to thirty minutes.

- Apple cider vinegar: Fights fatigue, relieves sunburn and itchy skin
- Bran: Softens skin and relieves itchiness
- Chamomile: Soothes skin and opens pores
- Epsom salts: Increases perspiration, relaxes muscles
- Ginger powder: Relaxes muscles, tones skin, increases circulation
- Jasmine flowers: Soothes the nerves
- Lavender: Relaxes muscles
- Lemon peel: Relieves muscle tension, stimulates the mind
- Nutmeg: Increases perspiration
- Oatmeal: Relieves itchiness, hives, sunburn
- Pine: Increases perspiration, softens skin, and relieves rashes
- Rosemary: Stimulates blood circulation
- Sage: Increases perspiration
- Salt: Soothes and relaxes muscles

While you are running the bath water, add about ½ cup of dried herbs to the water. (Be sure to cover the drain with a thin mesh screen or several layers of folded cheesecloth to filter out the herbs and prevent them from clogging the pipes.) For an Epsom salts bath, dissolve 2 pounds in the hot water. For essential oils, use a few drops of oil in the bath. For oatmeal, add 1 pound of uncooked oatmeal wrapped in a gauze bag. (Leave the bag in the water while you soak.)

CHAPTER ELEVEN

Other Complementary Treatments: From Quick Cures to Quackery

There's no arguing with success, but anecdotal evidence and impassioned testimonials are not enough for most health care professionals to recommend an unproven arthritis remedy. Keep in mind that unproven does not necessarily mean ineffective—but it also doesn't mean that the remedy has withstood rigorous testing for safety and efficacy.

To the medical community an arthritis treatment is considered safe and effective only after years of controlled clinical trials to prove that the treatment works for a significant number of patients without causing harmful side effects.

Of course critics claim that unproven remedies are nothing but a waste of money and energy. But arthritis sufferers often reach the point where they're willing to try *anything* to find relief. In fact some experts estimate that as many as 90 percent of people with arthritis eventually resort to unproven, unorthodox remedies to ease their pain. If you're searching for a cure for your arthritis pain and nothing else has worked, you may want to exercise caution but go ahead and give them a try as well.

While some measure of skepticism can be helpful in dealing with health care, remember that one year's quack cure is the next year's breakthrough cure, endorsed by the medical community. Consider that gold was first used in the treatment of rheumatoid arthritis in the 1920s. Though it effectively treated the condition in many patients, many doctors turned their backs on its use as an arthritis treatment because they didn't understand how it worked and because it suggested the disreputable practice of alchemy. Of course it is now in widespread use by even the most conservative physicians.

The line between orthodox treatment and quack cures is not always as clear as one might assume. Any health care practitioner or any treatment *promising* a cure should be looked at with caution, and anyone encouraging you to ignore your traditional medical care should also be avoided. But between conventional care and quackery lies a wide range of unproven—but possibly useful—treatments that may provide some measure of arthritis pain relief.

Balms, Ointments, and Topical Treatments

Some people find it soothing to rub their joints with analgesic lotions, liniments, oils, and gels enriched with camphor, menthol, or methyl salicylate. These treatments do nothing to reduce inflammation or treat the underlying arthritic condition, but they can bring temporary relief as a counterirritant, making the skin feel hot, cold, tingly, or numb.

If you want to give a topical treatment a try, look for one with a high percentage of methyl salicylate on the label. However, be aware that if you are allergic to aspirin or other salicylates, these products should be avoided since some of the active ingredients will be absorbed through the skin.

Chiropractic Manipulation

Some arthritis sufferers have placed themselves in the hands of chiropractors, who manipulate and adjust the vertebrae in the spine to remove pressure on the nerves and provide pain relief. The technique provides relief to some patients, but it aggravates pain for others.

The word *chiropractic* comes from the Greek words meaning "hand" and "done by." The technique was developed in 1895 by David Palmer (1845–1913), a Canadian healer who claims to have restored the hearing in a previously deaf man by manipulating his neck. Palmer developed his theory that human health was dependent on the flawless functioning of the nervous system; errant vertebrae in the spine could cause pressure on the nerves, which in turn caused pain and other health problems elsewhere in the body. In the terminology of chiropractic manipulation an impediment in the flow of nervous impulses is the result of "subluxation," or the misplacement of one or more vertebrae in the spine.

While some modern chiropractors continue to support the "single cause, single cure" approach, many others now embrace a holistic form of healing, which also takes into account the patient's overall health, including diet, nutritional supplements, relaxation techniques, and even psychotherapy.

Chiropractors use X rays and standard neurological tests to diagnose problems and dislocations of the spine. They cannot prescribe drugs or perform surgery; instead they correct or "adjust" the vertebrae, using dynamic thrusts to put the spine in correct alignment or more gentle manipulations to realign the joints.

For more information about chiropractors, contact the American Chiropractic Association, 1701 Clarendon Boulevard, Arlington, Virginia 22209; (800) 986-INFO or (703) 276-8800.

Copper Bracelets

Wearing a copper bracelet helps some arthritis sufferers ease the pain, though there is no objective scientific evidence that the bracelet treatment works. Studies have shown that some people with arthritis have difficulty metabolizing the copper found in the food they eat or the dietary supplements they take. This has led to the theory that the bracelet works by allowing the copper to be directly absorbed through the skin, bypassing the oral route.

DMSO

DMSO (dimethyl sulfoxide) is an unproven arthritis remedy with a devoted following, but one that should *not* be used. It is an industrial solvent similar to turpentine. In the 1960s scientists tested the drug as a possible treatment for a number of conditions, including rheumatoid arthritis, but researchers at the National Academy of Sciences concluded that the drug was ineffective and too dangerous to become a prescription drug for arthritis. A sterile form of DMSO, called Rimso-50, is used currently to treat a rare bladder condition, as well as by veterinarians to treat bruises in dogs and horses.

Flotation Tanks

After floating around in a sensory-deprivation tank (or flotation tank) for about an hour, many arthritis patients report a feeling of deep relaxation and significant pain relief. The water in the tanks is typically heated to 93.5 degrees F—the temperature of the skin—and the surrounding air is warm and still. This environment promotes relaxation and a feeling of tranquillity, which can ease the pain due to stress. For more information and a referral to a facility near you, contact the Floatation Tank Association, P.O. Box 1396, Grass Valley, California 95945; (916) 477-1319.

Lasers

Lasers are focused beams of light concentrated at specific wavelengths. When tightly controlled, these beams are powerful enough to cut diamonds and hot enough to cauterize bleeding tissue. The amount of heat can be altered by determining the length of time the beam is flashed, and it can be focused with surgical precision.

Surgeons routinely use lasers in eye surgery and other medical procedures, and some rheumatologists report benefits in treating rheumatoid arthritis. Currently the results are preliminary, but you may want to discuss the procedure with your rheumatologist if you're interested in learning more about it, or contact the American Society for Laser Medicine and Surgery, 2404 Stewart Square, Wausau, Wisconsin 54401; (715) 845-9283.

Reflexology

Reflexology is a specialized form of massage that involves stimulating the soles of the feet and hands in order to heal various parts of the body. The technique was developed in China and India at approximately the same time that acupuncture and acupressure were discovered.

Reflexology is based on the idea that the internal organs share the same nerve supplies as certain areas on the soles of the feet. (These points are not the same as those used in acupressure or acupuncture.) By pressing on certain points on the soles a practitioner of reflexology can stimulate organs throughout the body.

The technique, which was brought to the United States in the 1930s, has been growing in popularity, often with healers who also use chiropractic manipulation, homeopathy, and other methods of natural healing. During a reflexology session the patient lies on a massage table as the practitioner feels the feet for ''crystals,'' or waste deposits that build up in the nerve endings and restrict the flow of blood and nerve impulses. By massaging the area the practitioner breaks up the deposits, allowing them to be carried away.

For more information on reflexology, contact the International Institute of Reflexology, P.O. Box 12642, Saint Petersburg, Florida 33733; (813) 343-4811.

TENS

TENS—transcutaneous electrical nerve stimulation—uses low-level electrical charges to stimulate the nerves and block pain signals to the brain. During the treatment small electrodes are attached to the skin with a dab of gel to increase electrical conductivity. The electrodes are positioned at the relevant trigger points used in acupressure. On the other end the electrodes attach to a battery-operated box about the size of a pack of cigarettes, which releases low-level shocks just strong enough to cause a tingling sensation on the skin.

The success rate with TENS varies dramatically between patients; some people get no relief, whereas others report pain relief for hours or days. It is not clear whether the device works by altering the brain's perception of pain or by triggering the release of pain-killing endorphins.

A TENS device can be rented or purchased. The treatment is typically used only for chronic, local pain that fails to respond to other treatment. TENS should never be used by anyone with a pacemaker.

Yoga

Yoga is a form of exercise that focuses on mind-body unity. The technique involves moving the body into a series of postures, or positions, which promote relaxation. These movements also stretch and strengthen the muscles. (Many are similar or identical to the range-of-motion exercises many people with arthritis receive from their doctors and physical therapists.)

You don't have to be able to twist yourself into a number of seemingly uncomfortable positions to practice yoga. In fact the method is very gentle, noncompetitive, and non-threatening to beginners. Anyone can do yoga, though some people may be better than others at stretching and balancing. The postures are combined with deep breathing, relaxation techniques, and a healthful diet.

When practicing yoga, it is critical to exercise regularly. For best results practice yoga forty-five minutes a day. But even doing fifteen minutes a day is better than doing a longer session only once or twice a week.

For background on yoga postures and practicing the technique, get a book on yoga from your local library or take a class at a local Y or recreation facility. Or you could contact the Integral Yoga Institute, 227 West 13th Street, New York, New York 10011; (212) 929-0586.

Make Your Life a Little Easier

Arthritis can make the simplest task one of the day's greatest challenges. During a flare-up the toilet seat can seem too low, the telephone too difficult to dial, and a jar of strawberry preserves too stubborn to open.

Living with arthritis means enjoying the good days and enduring the bad. But there are specific steps you can take to simplify and improve the quality of your life—on both good days and bad.

- **Save your strength.** Pace yourself throughout the day so that you don't have to rush, strain, or overtire yourself trying to get everything done.
- **Get your house in order.** Reorganize your home and desk so that you can use your energy more efficiently. Keep cooking utensils near the stove; store the dishes near the dishwasher; store the common items you use at work within reach at your desk.
- **Give yourself a break.** Build short rest periods into your daily routine. Get up and stretch every half hour or so.
- **Focus on your body.** Be aware of how you hold yourself during the day. Avoid stooping. Sit up straight. Lift with your knees bent and your back straight to avoid back strain. (Or, better yet, slide an object rather than lifting it.) At work choose a chair with a firm back and good ergonomics. If you work at a desk, make sure it's two inches below your elbow height.
- **Take a load off.** Sit down whenever possible. Rest on a bar stool when working in the kitchen. If you can't avoid standing, shift your weight from one side to the other and take frequent breaks.
- **Bigger is better.** Whenever possible, use large joints and muscle groups rather than small ones, which can be more easily strained. For example use your hips and shoulders rather than your hands to push open a door.
- **Go easy on yourself.** Do what you can to take advantage of energy-saving devices and lifestyle changes that can make your life run more smoothly. However, before you reorder your life and rush out and buy every gadget that promises convenience, ask your doctor whether it would

be better for you to work through the pain and use your joints through various daily activities.

If the challenges of daily life aren't necessary for daily exercise, consider the following energy-saving tips:

- Use jar openers.
- Get a cart with wheels to move things from room to room.
- Install an elevated toilet seat, a bench in the bath, and a handrail in the tub.
- Use liquid soap instead of fighting with slippery bar soap.
- Choose clothes with front openings and elastic waists.
- Wear brassieres with front closures.
- Keep heavy objects at waist level to avoid stooping or reaching.
- Use an upright vacuum cleaner.
- Replace light switches with touch-sensitive switchplates.

ARTHRITIS RIP-OFF TIP-OFFS

Unfortunately quackery is common in the treatment of arthritis, in part because of the erratic symptoms associated with the illness. Quackery is big business; according to the U.S. Food and Drug Administration, health fraud costs Americans about $10 billion a year.

Protect yourself by looking for warning signs that a particular treatment, gadget, or procedure could be a waste of time and money. A report issued by the Council of Better Business Bureaus titled ''Arthritis: Quackery and Unproven Remedies'' offers the following suggestions:

- Be wary of guaranteed cures and promises of immediate and complete pain relief.
- Disregard the significance of testimonials from satisfied clients that cannot be independently verified. Testimonials should not replace scientific research as a proof of efficacy.
- Be suspicious of words such as *breakthrough, secret cure,* and *exclusive.* Hysterical language is not necessary to sell a product that works. Also any product with a "secret" formula is a scam. Scientists share their findings so that their work can be reviewed and verified. Important medical breakthroughs are not kept secret.
- Avoid taking advice from any service or practitioner that encourages you to distrust your physician or the Food and Drug Administration.
- Pass by any advertisement for a product that boasts of FDA approval. Federal law prohibits use of the agency name in any advertising that implies approval for a drug or medical device.
- Forget any product that promises to work on all types of arthritis. Arthritis refers to more than one hundred conditions, with many different treatments.
- Put your antennae up if an advertisement for a product boasts about a single study. Studies must be repeated to be considered valid.
- Don't buy a product that does not list the ingredients. Some miracle arthritis cures are nothing more than aspirin; others are dangerous and powerful drugs, such as corticosteroids. Find out what you're buying before you put your money down—and certainly before you consume any product.
- Red flag: No warning or mention of side effects. All treatments can have unintended effects, and it is the obligation of the seller to notify you of any potential hazards or inconveniences.

For more warning signs and information on medical quackery, contact the National Council Against Health Fraud, P.O. Box 1276, Loma Linda, California 92354-1276; (909) 824-4690.

CHAPTER TWELVE

Resources and Reading Lists

This book can provide an overview of natural remedies and therapies for arthritis, but you may want to know more about specific treatments for your particular problems. The following organizations on arthritis and natural medicine will help you track down the experts you need. Additional information is provided in the "Resources" sections in the rest of the book.

Resources

Arthritis

For free information on all types of arthritis, for physician and clinic referrals, or for the location of the Arthritis Foundation office in your area, contact:

The Arthritis Foundation
1314 Spring Street, N.W.
Atlanta, Georgia 30309
(404) 872-7100
(800) 283-7800

The National Institute of Arthritis and Musculoskeletal and
Skin Diseases coordinates the federal research on arthritis.
For more information on current medical research in the
area, contact:

**National Arthritis and Musculoskeletal and Skin
Diseases Information Clearinghouse**
9000 Rockville Pike
P.O. Box AMS
Bethesda, Maryland 20892-2903
(301) 495-4484

Rheumatology
The American College of Rheumatology, the professional
organization of rheumatologists, can provide a state-by-state
listing of certified rheumatologists. For more information,
contact:

American College of Rheumatology
60 Executive Park South
Suite 150
Atlanta, Georgia 30329
(404) 633-3777

Systemic Lupus Erythematosus
For more information about systemic lupus erythematosus,
contact:

L.E. Support Club (Lupus Erythematosus)
8039 Nova Court
North Charleston, South Carolina 29418
(803) 764-1769

Lupus Foundation of America
515-A East Braddock Road
Alexandria, Virginia 22302
(703) 684-2925

Lupus Network
230 Ranch Drive
Bridgeport, Connecticut 06606
(203) 372-5795

Ankylosing Spondylitis
For more information about ankylosing spondylitis, contact:

Ankylosing Spondylitis Association
511 North La Cienega
Suite 216
Los Angeles, Virginia 90048
(800) 777-8189

Juvenile Arthritis
For more information about juvenile arthritis, contact:

American Juvenile Arthritis Association
1314 Spring Street
Atlanta, Georgia 30309
(404) 872-7100

Scleroderma
For more information about scleroderma, contact:

Scleroderma Federation
Peabody Office Building
One Newbury Street
Peabody, Massachusetts 01960
(508) 535-6600

Scleroderma International Foundation
704 Gardner Center Road
New Castle, Pennsylvania 16101
(412) 652-3109

Scleroderma Research Foundation
P.O. Box 200
Columbus, New Jersey 08022
(609) 261-2200

United Scleroderma Foundation
P.O. Box 350
Watsonville, California 95077
(408) 728-2202

Naturopathy

Naturopathic physicians are graduates of a four-year post-graduate medical-sciences program. Their training includes courses in herbal medicine, nutrition, homeopathy, exercise therapy, acupressure, and acupuncture. In ten states—Alaska, Arizona, Connecticut, Florida, Hawaii, Montana, New Hampshire, Oregon, Utah, and Washington—naturopathic physicians (N.D.'s) must pass a state licensing exam.

For a directory of qualified naturopathic physicians, contact the professional organization of licensed naturopathic physicians:

The American Association of Naturopathic Physicians
2366 East Lake Avenue East, Suite 322
Seattle, Washington 98102
(206) 323-7610

There is a $5 fee for the information packet and national directory.

The Homeopathic Academy of Naturopathic Physicians
P.O. Box 69565
Portland, Oregon 97201
(503) 795-0579

The Council of Homeopathic Certification
1709 Seabright Avenue
Santa Cruz, California 95062
(408) 421-0565

Holistic Medicine

Holistic medicine is practiced by medical doctors (M.D.'s), osteopaths (D.O.'s), and naturopaths (N.D.'s). These physicians emphasize the treatment of the whole person and encourage personal responsibility for health.

For a national directory of licensed holistic practitioners, contact:

The American Holistic Medical Association
4101 Lake Boone Trail #201
Raleigh, North Carolina 26707
(919) 787-5146

There is an $8 fee for the information packet and national directory. The Association also publishes the magazine *Holistic Medicine* four times a year.

For information on courses and workshops on coping with chronic disease using holistic healing, contact:

Rise Institute
P.O. Box 2733
Petaluma, California 94973
(707) 765-2758

For information on physicians dedicated to holistic medical practices, contact:

Center for Mind-Body Medicine
5225 Connecticut Avenue, N.W.
Suite 414
Washington, DC 20015
(202) 966-7338

Reading Lists

Books on Arthritis
Arthritis Alternatives by Irna and Laurence Gadd (New York: Warner Books, 1985).

The Arthritis Helpbook by Kate Loring, R.N., and James F. Fries, M.D. (Reading, Mass.: Addison-Wesley, 1980).

Arthritis: How You Can Benefit from Diet, Vitamins, Minerals, Herbs, Exercise, and Other Natural Methods by Michael T. Murray, N.D. (Rocklin, Calif.: Prima Publishing, 1994).

Arthritis Relief at Your Fingertips: Your Guide to Easing Aches and Pains Without Drugs by Michael Reed Gach (New York: Warner Books, 1989).

Arthritis: Relief Beyond Drugs by Rachel Carr (New York: Harper & Row, 1981).

The Arthritis Sourcebook by Earl J. Brewer, Jr., M.D., and Kathy Cochran Angel (Los Angeles: RGA Publishing Group, 1993).

Arthritis: What Works by Dava Sobel and Arthur C. Klein (New York: St. Martin's, 1989).

Duke University Medical Center Book of Arthritis by David S. Pisetsky, M.D., Ph.D., with Susan Flamholtz Trien (New York: Fawcett Columbine, 1992).

A Natural Approach: Arthritis by Michio Kushi (New York: Japan Publications, Inc, 1988).

Relief from Chronic Arthritis Pain by Helene MacLean (New York: Dell, 1990).

Understanding Arthritis by the Arthritis Foundation (New York: Scribner's, 1984).

Books on Natural Medicine

Acupressure for Everybody by Cathryn Bauer (New York: Henry Holt and Co., 1991).

Acupressure's Potent Points by Michael Reed Gach (New York: Bantam Books, 1990).

Acupuncture: How It Works, How It Cures by Peter Firebrace and Sandra Hill (New Canaan, Conn.: Keats Publishing Inc., 1994).

A to Z Guide to Healing Herbal Remedies by Jason Elias, M.A., and Shelagh Ryan Masline (New York: Dell, 1995).

The Complete Guide to Vitamins, Minerals, Supplements, and Herbs by Winter H. Griffith (Tuscon, Ariz.: Fisher Books, 1988).

The Concise Herbal Encyclopedia by Donald Law (New York: St. Martin's Press, 1973).

The Encyclopedia of Alternative Health Care by Kristin Gottschalk Olsen (New York: Pocket Books, 1989).

Encyclopedia of Natural Medicine by Michael Murray, N.D., and Joseph Pizzorono, N.D. (Rocklin, Calif.: Prima Publishing, 1991).

The Food Pharmacy by Jean Carper (New York: Bantam Books, 1988).

Food—Your Miracle Medicine: How Food Can Prevent and Cure Over 100 Symptoms and Problems by Jean Carper (New York: HarperCollins, 1993).

Growing and Using the Healing Herbs by Gaea and Shandor Weiss (Emmaus, Pa.: Rodale Press, 1985).

The Healing Herbs: The Ultimate Guide to the Curative Power of Nature's Medicines by Michael Castleman (New York: Bantam Books, 1991).

Health and Healing by Andrew Weil, M.D. (Boston: Houghton Mifflin Co., 1983).

Herbal Healing by Michael Hallowell (Garden City Park, N.Y.: Avery Publishing Group, 1994).

The Honest Herbal by Varro Tyler, Ph.D. (Binghamton, N.Y.: Pharmaceutical Products Press, 1993).

Macrobiotic Diet by Michio and Aveline Kushi (New York: Japan Publications, 1985).

The Macrobiotic Way by Michio Kushi and Stephen Blauer (Avery Publishing Group, 1985).

Magic and Medicine of Plants edited by Inge N. Dobelis (Pleasantville, N.Y.: Reader's Digest, 1986).

Natural Health, Natural Medicine by Andrew Weil (Boston: Houghton Mifflin, 1990).

The Natural Pharmacy Product Guide by Richard Israel (Garden City Park, N.Y.: Avery Publishing Group, 1991).

Prescription for Nutritional Healing by James and Phyllis Balch (Garden City Park, N.Y.: Avery Publishing Group, 1990).

Reader's Digest Family Guide to Natural Medicine: How to Stay Healthy the Natural Way by The Reader's Digest Association, edited by Alma E. Guinness (New York: Reader's Digest, 1993).

Rodale's Illustrated Encyclopedia of Herbs edited by Claire Kowalchik and William H. Hylton (Emmaus, Pa.: Rodale Press, 1987).

Glossary

ALLOPURINOL: A drug used to treat gout attacks by blocking the formation of uric acid.

ANALGESIC: A class of drugs used to relieve pain.

ANKYLOSING SPONDYLITIS: A type of arthritis involving the spine and sacroiliac joints. The condition begins with inflammation of the tendons and ligaments where they attach to the spine; in later stages the bones in the spine may fuse together.

ANTINUCLEAR ANTIBODY (ANA): Antibodies found in people with many types of connective-tissue disease, including rheumatoid arthritis, lupus, and scleroderma.

ARTHRITIS: The term for a group of more than one hundred rheumatic diseases affecting the joints, muscles, tendons, ligaments, and other connective tissues.

ARTHROCENTESIS: A medical procedure that involves inserting a hollow needle into a joint to withdraw a sample of synovial fluid.

ARTHROPLASTY: Surgical joint reconstruction; most arthroplasties involve total joint replacement with a prosthesis, though reconstruction can also be done using the patient's own tissues.

AUTOIMMUNE DISEASE: A medical condition in which the immune system malfunctions and the body attacks its own tissue.

BOUCHARD'S NODES: Bony enlargements or growths on the middle joints of the fingers; the nodes can be symptoms of osteoarthritis.

BURSA: A fibrous, fluid-filled pouch that reduces friction and cushions the areas between the bones and muscles. The fluid allows the bones, tendons, and muscles to glide smoothly over each other.

BURSITIS: Inflammation of the bursa.

CARTILAGE: Tough, elastic tissue that covers and cushions the ends of the bones where joints are formed.

COLCHICINE: A drug used in the treatment of gout.

COLLAGEN: A protein component of bones and connective tissues, including cartilage, skin, and tendons.

CONNECTIVE TISSUE: The ligaments, tendons, and muscles throughout the body that attach to the bones and form the framework of the body and the internal organs.

CONTRACTURE: A type of joint deformity resulting in loss of joint flexibility and shortening of the connective tissues. The joint can lose its range of motion or become locked. (Also called flexion contracture.)

CORTICOSTEROIDS: Drugs that quickly reduce swelling and inflammation; they can either be produced by the adrenal cortex or synthetically made.

CORTISONE: An example of a corticosteroid.

CPPD DISEASE: A type of arthritis caused by the deposit of calcium pyrophosphate dihydrate crystals (CPPD) in the joints, sometimes referred to as pseudogout.

ERYTHROCYTE SEDIMENTATION RATE (ESR): A diagnostic test involving the measurement of how quickly red blood cells drop to the bottom of a test tube filled with whole blood. Red blood cells (erythrocytes) fall faster in the presence of inflammation, common with rheumatoid arthritis.

FIBROSITIS: Pain and inflammation of the connective tissues. (Also called muscle rheumatism.)

FLARE-UP: A period when arthritic symptoms reemerge or intensify.

GENETIC MARKER: A specific tissue type passed down through the genes. There is a link between certain genetic markers and certain types of arthritis.

GOUT: A type of arthritis characterized by the deposit of monosodium urate crystals in the joints, especially the big toe.

HEBERDEN'S NODES: Bony growths on the finger joints nearest the fingertip in patients with osteoarthritis.

HUMAN LEUKOCYTE ANTIGENS (HLA): Genetic markers associated with increased risk of developing certain types of arthritis. HLA-B27 has been linked to a predisposition to develop ankylosing spondylitis and Reiter's syndrome; HLA-DR4 has been linked to rheumatoid arthritis.

HYPERURICEMIA: A medical condition characterized by high levels of uric acid in the blood. The condition is not diagnostic of gout; it can be associated with kidney dysfunction or the use of diuretics.

IMMUNE SYSTEM: The system of defenses used by the body to protect itself from disease, infection, or injury.

INFLAMMATION: The body's reaction to injury, infection, or disease characterized by swelling, redness, heat, and pain.

JOINT: The junction where two bones meet.

JUVENILE ARTHRITIS: The term used to describe a number of types of arthritis when they occur in children.

LIGAMENT: A band of tough, cordlike tissue that connects one bone to another.

LYME DISEASE: A bacterial disease caused by a deer-tick bite. If not promptly treated with antibiotics, the disease can cause joint inflammation and arthritic symptoms.

NONSTEROIDAL ANTIINFLAMMATORY DRUGS (NSAIDS): A group of drugs that relieve pain and reduce inflammation. Examples include aspirin, ibuprofen, naproxen, and indomethacin, among others.

OSSIFICATION: The process of turning soft tissue into hard, bonelike substances. Ossification may cause the spine to become rigid in people with ankylosing spondylitis.

OSTEOARTHRITIS: A degenerative form of arthritis caused by damage to the cartilage, sometimes caused by excessive wear and tear on the joints.

OSTEOPHYTE: Small bonelike growth at the end of the bones where cartilage has been worn away by osteoarthritis. (Also known as spurs.)

PAUCIARTICULAR DISEASE: A type of arthritis that affects only a few joints, especially in children.

POLYARTICULAR DISEASE: A type of arthritis that affects five or more joints. The term is often used to describe a form of juvenile arthritis that is similar to adult rheumatoid arthritis.

PROSTAGLANDINS: Hormonelike substances produced by the body; inhibiting the action of some prostaglandins boosts the effectiveness of antiinflammatory drugs.

PSEUDOGOUT: A type of arthritis caused by crystal deposits of calcium pyrophosphate dihydrate (CPPD); the condition is similar to gout, but can be treated with nonsteroidal antiinflammatory drugs. Pseudogout commonly affects the knees.

RAYNAUD'S PHENOMENON: A type of arthritis that involves extreme fluctuations in temperature of the fingers and toes in response to cold or emotional upset. Changes in the small blood vessels can cause sensations of burning, tingling, and numbness.

REITER'S SYNDROME: A type of arthritis that sometimes follows gastrointestinal, genital, or urinary-tract infections. Joint inflammation, especially in the knees and ankles, may follow two to six weeks after the original infection. (Also known as reactive arthritis.)

RESECTION: A surgical procedure to remove damaged bone from a joint to relieve pain.

RHEUMATOID ARTHRITIS: A chronic disease characterized by pain, stiffness, swelling, and inflammation of the joints throughout the body.

RHEUMATOID FACTOR: An antibody often found in people with rheumatoid arthritis.

RHEUMATOLOGIST: A physician who specializes in the treatment of rheumatic diseases.

SALICYLISM: A condition caused by high doses of drugs containing salicylates, such as aspirin. Symptoms include ringing in the ears (tinnitus), hearing loss, confusion, irritability, and abnormal breathing.

SCLERODERMA: A rare form of arthritis involving the production of excessive amounts of collagen.

SYNOVECTOMY: A surgical procedure to remove the diseased joint lining or synovium.

SYNOVIAL FLUID: A thick, clear gel produced by the synovial membrane to lubricate the joints.

SYNOVIAL MEMBRANE (SYNOVIUM): The thin lining that surrounds the inside of the joints.

SYSTEMIC LUPUS ERYTHEMATOSUS: A type of arthritis that affects the skin, muscles, and joints; in some cases it also affects the internal organs.

TENDONS: Tough bands of tissue that connect muscle to bone.

URIC ACID: A waste product resulting from the chemical breakdown of purines in the body; excessive amounts of uric acid in the blood can lead to the formation of crystals, which collect in the joints and cause gout.

Index

About the Authors

Winifred Conkling comes from a long line of medical professionals. Her great-great-grandfather was a physician who sent his three
sons through three different types of medical training: one became a
homeopath, the second an allopath, and the third a naturopath. After
medical school the brothers practiced medicine together, sharing
their knowledge for the benefit of their patients. Since then every
generation has included at least one physician; both of Conkling's
parents were medical doctors.

Conkling is a freelance writer specializing in health and consumer topics. She is the author of *Natural Healing for Children* (St.
Martin's, 1996) and *Securing Your Child's Future: A Financial and
Legal Planner for Parents* (Ballantine, 1995); and she is working on
the upcoming book *Stop the Clock! Natural Remedies for Aging*
(Dell, 1997). She has also written several other books, and her work
has been published in a number of national magazines. She lives in
northern Virginia with her husband and two children.

Andrea D. Sullivan, PhD, ND, DHANP, received a degree in naturopathic medicine from Bastyr University in Seattle. She is a
Diplomate of the Homeopathic Academy of Naturopathic Physicians and a frequent speaker at professional conferences and semi-
nars. She practices in Washington, D.C., and is at work on her book,
*Naturopathic Medicine for African-Americans: A Choice for
Health,* to be published by Anchor Books in 1997.